SpringerBriefs in Computer Science

More information about this series at http://www.springer.com/series/10028

Juris Klonovs • Mohammad A. Haque
Volker Krueger • Kamal Nasrollahi
Karen Andersen-Ranberg • Thomas B. Moeslund
Erika G. Spaich

Distributed Computing and Monitoring Technologies for Older Patients

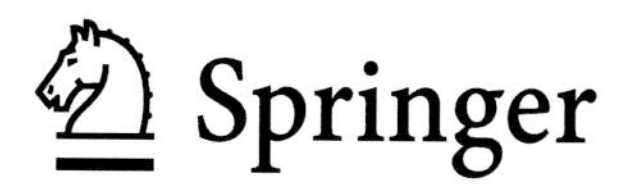

Juris Klonovs
M-Tech
Aalborg University
Copenhagen, Denmark

Volker Krueger
Aalborg University
Copenhagen, Denmark

Karen Andersen-Ranberg
Danish Aging Research Center
University of Southern Denmark
Odense, Denmark

Erika G. Spaich
Department of Health Science
and Technology
Aalborg University
Aalborg, Denmark

Mohammad A. Haque
Architecture, Design, & Media Technology
Aalborg University
Aalborg, Denmark

Kamal Nasrollahi
Architecture, Design & Media Technology
Aalborg University
Aalborg, Denmark

Thomas B. Moeslund
Visual Analysis of People Lab
Aalborg University
Aalborg, Denmark

ISSN 2191-5768 ISSN 2191-5776 (electronic)
SpringerBriefs in Computer Science
ISBN 978-3-319-27023-4 ISBN 978-3-319-27024-1 (eBook)
DOI 10.1007/978-3-319-27024-1

Library of Congress Control Number: 2015960745

Springer Cham Heidelberg New York Dordrecht London

Printed on acid-free paper

Springer International Publishing AG Switzerland is part of Springer Science+Business Media (www.springer.com)

Preface

In this book, we summarize recently deployed monitoring approaches with a focus on automatically detecting health threats for older patients living alone at home. First, in order to give an overview of the problems at hand, we briefly describe older adults who would mostly benefit from healthcare supervision and explain their potential health threats and dangerous situations, which need to be detected timely. Second, we summarize possible scenarios for monitoring an older patient at home and derive common functional requirements for monitoring technology. Third, we identify the realistic state-of-the-art technological monitoring approaches, which are practically applicable to older adults, in general, and to geriatric patients, in particular. In order to uncover the majority of applicable solutions, we survey the interdisciplinary fields of smart homes, telemonitoring, ambient intelligence, ambient assisted living, gerotechnology, and aging-in-place technology among others. Consequently, we discuss the related experimental studies and how they collect and analyze the measured data, focusing on the application of sensor fusion, signal processing, and machine learning techniques whenever possible, which are shown to be useful for improving the detection and identification of situations that can threaten older adults' health. Finally, we discuss future challenges and offer a number of suggestions for further research directions. We conclude the book by highlighting the open issues within automatic healthcare technologies and link them to potential solutions.

Keywords: eHealth, Telemonitoring, Home care, Smart homes, Ambient intelligence (AmI), Ambient assisted living (AAL), Machine learning, Sensors, Geriatric conditions

Copenhagen, Denmark — Juris Klonovs
Aalborg, Denmark — Mohammad A. Haque
Copenhagen, Denmark — Volker Krueger
Aalborg, Denmark — Kamal Nasrollahi
Odense, Denmark — Karen Andersen-Ranberg
Aalborg, Denmark — Thomas B. Moeslund
Aalborg, Denmark — Erika G. Spaich

Acknowledgments

The writing of this book was supported by the Innovation Fund Denmark and Growth Forum in the Region of Southern Denmark through the project Patient@home.

Contents

Abbreviations

AAL	Ambient Assisted Living
ADLs	Activities of Daily Living
AI	Artificial Intelligence
ALT	Assisted Living Technology
AmI	Ambient Intelligence
ANN	Artificial Neural Network
ARBF	Augmented Radial Basis Function
AT	Assistive Technology
BP	Blood Pressure
CAM	Confusion Assessment Method
CEN	European Committee for Standardization
CGA	Comprehensive Geriatric Assessment
CHD	Coronary Heart Disease
COPD	Chronic Obstructive Pulmonary Diseases
CRF	Conditional Random Field
DBN	Dynamic Bayesian Network or Deep Belief Network (Depending on Context)
DS	Danish Standard
DTs	Decision Trees
ECG	Electrocardiography
EEG	Electroencephalography
EHR	Electronic Health Records
EMG	Electromyography
EN	European Norms
EU	European Union
FP7	Seventh Framework Programme
FVC	Forced Vital Capacity
GMM	Gaussian Mixture Models
GPs	Gaussian Processes

GPS	Global Positioning System
GSM	Global System for Mobile Communications
GSR	Galvanic Skin Response
HH	Hospital at Home
HMMs	Hidden Markov Models
HR	Heart Rate
HRV	Heart Rate Variability
IADL	Instrumental Activity of Daily Living
ICT	Information and Communication Technologies
IEC	International Electrotechnical Commission
IP	Internet Protocol or Impedance Pneumography (Depending on Context)
IR	Infrared
IRDA	Infrared Data Association
ISDN	Integrated Services for Digital Network
ISO	International Organization for Standardization
IT	Information Technology
kNN	k-Nearest Neighbor (Classifier)
MEDDEV	Medical Devices
NBC	Naïve Bayesian Classifier
NBN	Naïve Bayesian Network
NIRS	Near-Infrared Sensors
PDMS	Patient Data Management System
PEF	Peak Expiratory Flow
PIF	Peak Inspiratory Flow
PIR	Passive Infrared (Sensor)
PSTN	Public Switched Telephone Network
PTZ	Pan-Tilt-Zoom (Camera)
QoL	Quality of Life
QoS	Quality of Service
RF	Radio-Frequency
RFID	Radio-Frequency Identification
RGB	Red-Green-Blue
RGB-D	Red-Green-Blue Depth
SH	Smart Home
SVM	Support Vector Machine
TRF	Test Report Forms
UTI	Urinary Tract Infection
WBASN	Wireless Body Area Sensor Network
WHO	World Health Organization
WLAN	Wireless Local Area Network
WSN	Wireless Sensor Network

Chapter 1
Introduction

Abstract In recent years, distributed computing and monitoring technologies have gained a lot of interest in the cross-disciplinary field of healthcare informatics. This introductory chapter reveals the growing need for timely detection of numerous health threats of older people, who are challenged by various chronic and acute illnesses and are susceptible to injuries. First, we give a concise overview of the relevant terms, which are often used for representing state-of-the-art technologies and research fields dealing with monitoring of older patients. Second, we guide the readers through the contents of this book, which are intended for both geriatric care practitioners and engineers, who are developing or integrating monitoring solutions for older adults. Then, we provide a summary of notable worldwide smart-home projects aimed at monitoring and assisting older people, including geriatric patients. The underlying aim of these projects was to explore the use of ambient and/or wearable sensing technology to monitor the well-being of older adults in their home environments.

Keywords Geriatric patient • Elderly • Older adults • Automatic health monitoring • Smart-home • Patient at home • Telemonitoring • Assisted living • Gerotechnology • Caregiver • eHealth • Ambient intelligence (AmI) • Ambient assisted living (AAL)

Due to the changing demographics in most industrialized countries, the number and the proportion of older adults are rapidly increasing [1–3]. The risk of having to face health problems increases with advancing age. Advancing age is also associated with an increased risk of living alone and with having a potentially smaller social network [4]. Living alone also means having no supervision or proper care when needed, e.g., in case of a disease or an adverse event [5]. Timely detection of *health threats*[1] at home can be beneficial in numerous ways; for example, it can enable independence and can potentially reduce the need of institutionalization [6], facilitating so-called *aging-in-place* paradigm [7–9], which is defined as "the ability to

---

[1] In this book, we define a *health threat* as any possible health-threatening situation, condition, or risk factor, including external, such as environmental hazards, or internal, such as evolving diseases, as well as dangerous and life-threatening occurrences, such as falls or medication misuse.

J. Klonovs et al., *Distributed Computing and Monitoring Technologies for Older Patients*, SpringerBriefs in Computer Science,
DOI 10.1007/978-3-319-27024-1_1

live in one's own home and community safely, independently, and comfortably, regardless of age, income, or ability level" [10].

Eventually, when facing health problems, many older adults may prefer to stay in their own home, often due to the fear of losing the ability of managing their private life or possibility of being involved in their social relationships [11, 12]. Researchers argue that older adults who are staying at home with an appropriate assistance have a higher likelihood of staying healthy and independent longer [3, 13]. For example, there is evidence that older adults may experience significantly higher risk of becoming delirious at a hospital than at home [14]. For this and other reasons, geriatric patients should, in principle, be sent from a hospital to their home as quickly as possible. Consequently, this raises several challenges associated with the necessity of intensive monitoring by home care staff, which may be inadequate and privacy intrusive, to avoid further aggravation but secure recovery [15]. On the other hand, for those older adults, who are mobile and independent but at risk of the consequences of aging, early detection of deteriorating health is also essential for avoiding the necessity of hospitalization and eventually move to a nursing home. As a solution, in-home monitoring technology, if applied properly, can nowadays be used on both healthy older adults, for detecting health-threatening situations, and geriatric patients, for detecting adverse events or health deterioration. Therefore, there is a vastly growing interest in developing robust unobtrusive ubiquitous home-based health monitoring systems and services that can help older home dwellers to live safely and independently [16]. However, due to the high variety of possible scenarios and circumstances, keeping track on health conditions of an older individual at home may be exceedingly difficult.

In this book, we are looking for (a) *which* health threats should be detected, (b) *what* data is relevant for detecting these health threats, and (c) *how* to acquire the right data about an older home dweller. In particular, (a) and (b) include a proper understanding of the problems at hand, the possible constraints, and the needs seen by patients and medical staff, while (c) includes a choice of sensors and their placement. Furthermore, (a), (b), and (c) are closely interrelated. Then, we aim to uncover which approaches can automate detection of the health threats and extraction of relevant information and knowledge for supporting further decision-making.

In the past 15 years, a great number of monitoring technologies, which can gather patient-specific data automatically, have been developed to monitor and support frail older adults at home. The application of these technologies have become increasingly popular mainly due to the rapid advances in both sensor and information and communication technologies (ICT). They allow reduction of chronic disease complications and better follow-up, allow accessing healthcare services without using hospital beds, and reduce patient travel, time off from work, and overall costs [17]. Automated monitoring systems, which are becoming cheaper and less intrusive with each year, have been made possible for clinical use by reducing the size and cost of monitoring sensors, as well as of recording and transmitting hardware [18]. These hardware developments, coupled with the available wired (e.g., PSTN, ISDN, IP)[2] and wireless (e.g., IrDA, WLAN, GSM)[3] telecommunication options, have led to the development of various home monitoring applications. For the deployment of these kinds of technologies, several terms have been coined, such as *smart-home* [19–25], *home automation* [19, 23, 25–28], *ubiquitous home* [24, 29–31], *ambient intelligence* (*AmI*) [32–37], *assistive technology* [38–40], *assisted living technology* (*ALT*) [41–43], *ambient assisted living* (*AAL*) [33, 34, 37, 44–49], *home telehealth* [50–52], *telemonitoring* [18, 50, 53–55], *wireless body area sensor networks* (*WBASNs*) [56–60], *aging-in-place* technologies [8, 9, 61], *gero(n)technology* [39, 62–64], *eHealth* [65, 66], and others. All these technologies are related (e.g., all incorporate *sensor technology*); however, each of them usually has diverse aims, and they can be supplementary to each other in terms of contributing to the monitoring purposes of older patients at home.

The schematic overlap of these most notable technological research areas is illustrated in Fig. 1.1. As it becomes evident, investigating automated monitoring of older patients with comorbidities at home requires us to understand and recognize the different related fields. Thus, definitions of these research fields along with discussion of relevance to this book are presented in the next chapter.

1.1 Definition of Terms and Relevance to This Book

The term *smart-home* has many diverse definitions [19–25]. A *smart-home* is often defined as a residence equipped with technology that observes its inhabitants and provides proactive services [21]. Most commonly, it refers to *home automation* [19, 23, 25–28], which by definition tackles four main goals: comfort, security, life safety, and low cost [28]. In the context of this book, we focus our analysis primarily on improving life safety, which is achieved by incorporating *telemonitoring* technology that can be a part of a *smart-home* as well.

Telemonitoring is originally defined as the use of audio, video, and other telecommunications and electronic information processing technologies to monitor patient status at a distance [67]. Thus, all the other systems intended for increasing the comfort of home inhabitants by automating their tasks or controlling home appliances (e.g., automatic light switches, dish washers, etc.) as well as energy management systems intended for reducing costs (e.g., by preventing unnecessary heating and lighting) do not fall into the scope of our book. It is also worth noting that the term *telemonitoring* is often used in different contexts, and thus, one should be very careful in identifying the methods of data collection and communication chosen for remote patient monitoring. Often in literature, manual self-reporting of health status via telephone (e.g., in [68]) is already considered as *telemonitoring*.

[2] *PSTN* – Public Switched Telephone Network; *ISDN* – Integrated Services for Digital Network; *IP* – Internet Protocol.

[3] *IRDA* – Infrared Data Association; *WLAN* – Wireless Local Area Network; *GSM* – Global System for Mobile Communications.

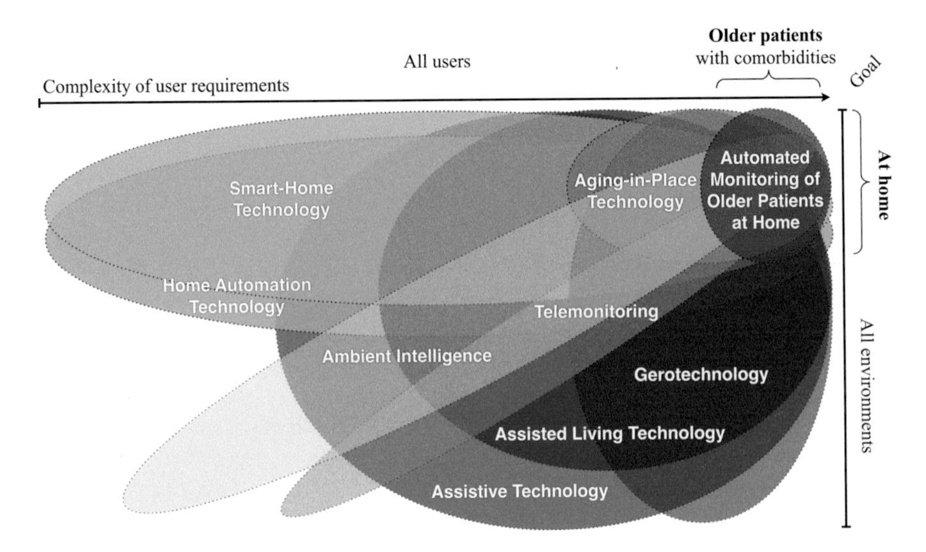

Fig. 1.1 An overlap of the most notable and emerging state-of-the-art technological research fields that contribute to automated monitoring of older patients at home. In this graph, we focus only on those technological domains, which explicitly or implicitly facilitate patient-centered care. Other related areas, such as ICT, wireless sensor networks, telematics, sensor fusion, machine learning, software engineering, etc. (purely from a technological point of view) and homecare, telehealth, telecare, telemedicine, mobile health (i.e., mHealth), etc. (which already indicate a healthcare point of view), are not visualized for redundancy reasons. The *horizontal axis* abstracts the domain of user requirements, while the *vertical axis* encapsulates the variety of different environments. Generally, the requirements of monitoring older patients at home are very complex, and thus a very limited selection of all possible technological advances can be practically useful for monitoring this target group. Hence, we schematically illustrate the applicability of the existing state-of-the-art monitoring technologies for geriatric patients at home as a *red oval* in the *upper right* corner of the figure

Meanwhile, numerous other automated information and communication technology (*ICT*) options exist in *telemonitoring*, enabling automatic and preferably more reliable data collection and transmission from home, which therefore are of interest for our book. For example, Paré et al. in their systematic review [55] defined the term *home telemonitoring* as an automated process for the transmission of data on a patient's health status from home to the respective healthcare setting. However, one should notice that this definition does not imply that data collection is also automated. They further explained that only patients, when necessary, are responsible for keying in and transmitting their data without the help of a healthcare provider, such as a nurse or a physician. However, since we are also interested in monitoring technologies, which might require healthcare provider being present and being responsible for acquiring the right data at a patient's home (e.g., during their homecare visits), our scope is not limited to *home telemonitoring* alone.

Health smart-home (HSH) [22, 24, 69, 70] is another relevant term derived from the marriage of *smart-home* technology and *medicine. HSH* is defined as a residence equipped with automatic devices and various sensors to ensure the safety of a patient at home and the supervision of their health status [71], which fits well with the focus of this book. *HSH* is a specialization of the general *smart-home* concept, which integrates sensors and actuators to ensure a medical *telemonitoring* to residents and to assist them in performing their activities of daily living (*ADL*) [22]. It also facilitates an *aging-in-place* process [22], because it aims at giving an autonomous life to older people in their own home, thus avoiding or postponing the need for institutional care.

Following the rapidly increasing deployment of wireless sensing devices, such devices have a growing impact on the way we live, and they open up possibilities to many healthcare applications that were not feasible previously. For maximizing the value of collected data, *wireless sensor networks* (*WSN*), *ubiquitous/pervasive computing*, and *artificial intelligence* (AI) as individual research domains have come together to build an interdisciplinary concept of *ambient intelligence* or *AmI* [35, 72]. The definition of *AmI*, however, is highly variable [34, 35, 73]. Most commonly, *AmI* is described as an emerging discipline that brings intelligence to everyday environments and makes those environments sensitive, adaptive, and responsive to human needs [32, 34, 35]. In addition, several studies require that *AmI* systems should be transparent (i.e., unobtrusive) [35, 74] and ubiquitous (i.e., present everywhere anytime) [32, 34, 35, 73, 74]. All this correlates well with the general requirements for *aging-in-place* technologies [8, 9] and *gerotechnology* [62], because these systems should be able to adopt to the needs of older adults, to sense hazardous or unsafe situations with minimal human intervention, and to inform a medical personnel and/or family members if something is truly “wrong” [9]. While *smart-home*, *home automation*, *ubiquitous home*, and *ambient intelligence* technologies can be intended for any user group and irrespective of age, *gerotechnology* is explicitly focusing on older adults, including older patients with comorbidities, while *aging-in-place* technology limits the deployment of the *gerotechnology* to private homes. *Aging-in-place* technology is a popular and a relatively general term, which refers to increasing the ability of older adults to stay in their own home as they age [75, 76], and is recognized as a part of *gerotechnology* (which is consequently derived from combination of two words: gerontology and technology). *Gerotechnology* plays a crucial role in the *aging-in-place* process and is defined as “an interdisciplinary field of research and application involving gerontology, the scientific study of aging, and technology, the development and distribution of technologically based products, environments, and services” [77]. However, *gerotechnology* does not necessarily involve intelligence in the sense of being sensitive and adjustable to patient’s needs. Different aging-associated aids (e.g., vision and hearing aids [78], or even walking aids [79] and toileting aids [80]) are often considered as appliances of *gerotechnology*; however, these do not directly fall into the scope of our book, unless they are capable of collecting meaningful medically relevant data, which we will reveal in the further chapters.

Most commonly, when dealing with geriatric or disabled patients, a majority of the aforementioned technologies employ *assistive technology* (*AT*), which by definition serves three major purposes relevant to life safety of patients at home [81]: (1) detecting hazards or emergencies, (2) facilitating independence and improving functional performance, and (3) supporting medical staff (i.e., caregivers) by facilitating provision of personal care. For our book, the main focus is put on the first purpose. One of the most important aspects that can differentiate *ATs* from other technologies is the *user-centered design*, which can be achieved by complying with numerous requirements defined by both medical and technical factors. Generally, it is considered to be a good practice to comply with *universal design* principles (often called as *design for all*) [82]. These fundamental principles include [82] (a) usage equitability, i.e., the design should be useful and marketable to people with diverse abilities; (b) flexibility in use, i.e., the design accommodates a wide range of individual preferences and abilities; (c) simple and intuitive use, i.e., easy to understand regardless of experience, knowledge, language skills, or current concentration level of the user; (d) perceptible information, i.e., the design communicates necessary information effectively to the user despite ambient conditions or sensory abilities of the user; (e) tolerance for error, i.e., the design minimizes hazards and the adverse consequences of accidental or unintended actions; (f) low physical effort, i.e., effective and comfortable usage with minimum of fatigue; and finally (g) size and space for approach and use, i.e., appropriate size and space should be provided for approach, reach, manipulation, and use regardless of human body size, posture, or mobility of a user, such as older patient.

Assisted living technologies (*ALTs*) is another relevant and broad term, which often remains undefined and may have different meanings throughout *aging-in-place* related literature [43]. Commonly, it refers to sensors, devices, and communication systems (including software), which, in combination, help to assist older adults and those who are physically or cognitively impaired in accomplishing their daily tasks toward independent lives and an improved quality of life, by delivering *assisted living services* [83, 84]. These services may include *telehealth services* (i.e., delivering medical care, treatment, and monitoring services at home from a remote location), *telecare services* (i.e., delivering social care and related monitoring services at home from a remote location), *wellness services* (i.e., delivering services for healthy lifestyles at home from a remote location), *digital participation services* (i.e., which remotely engage older and disabled people in terms of social, educational, or entertainment activities at home), and *teleworking services* (i.e., in which older and disabled people work remotely from home for an employer, a voluntary organization, or themselves and need remote computing to work successfully) [84]. Noteworthy, *telemedicine services* (i.e., which involve delivering medical services and advices from one practitioner to another at a remote location) are not considered to be a part of *ALTs* [84].

Assisted living technologies based on *ambient intelligence* are called *ambient assisted living* (*AAL*) *tools* [33], and they are, respectively, broader than our scope of monitoring and detecting health-threatening problems. *AAL* in general can be used for preventing health problems, treatment, and improving health conditions and well-being of older individuals. These tools can be installed in (*health*) *smart-homes* and therefore can greatly support monitoring purposes by collecting contextual information and recording *activities of daily living* (*ADL*) [85–88], for example. *ADL* may include any activity, which can be observed in daily living of an individual (e.g., walking, lying, and sitting, which are considered as basic activities, or preparing a coffee, laundering, cooking meals, and shopping groceries, which are considered as instrumental activities). A huge number of *AAL* tools exists, such as medication management tools [55, 89, 90], fall detection [91–95] and prevention systems [96–98], video surveillance systems [6, 99–101], indoor location tracking [102, 103], communication systems [8, 104, 105], mobile emergency response systems [8, 63, 106–108], and diet suggestion systems [109], which in general can be built and implemented with the purpose of health monitoring and improving safety, connectivity, and mobility of older adults at home.

The term *eHealth*, which nowadays seems to serve public as a general "buzzword," is currently defined by World Health Organization (WHO) as "the use of information and communication technologies (ICT) for health. Examples include treating patients, conducting research, educating the health workforce, tracking diseases and monitoring public health" [65]. In the light of this definition, our book is focused on tracking diseases and monitoring public health for older adult users. Apparently, definitions of *eHealth* seem to vary with respect to the functions, stakeholders, contexts, and various theoretical issues targeted [110]. The medical subject heading (MeSH) [111] library directly relates *eHealth* to the term *telemedicine*, which is defined as a "delivery of health services via remote telecommunications. This includes interactive consultative and diagnostic services." One may by intuition anticipate that *eHealth* refers to "electronic" healthcare, because of the prefix "e." However, the meaning of the letter "e" is rather ambiguous, and therefore, *eHealth* term can be found in a very broad context. Furthermore, *eHealth* and *E-Health* are often used interchangeably and considered as synonyms [110]. However, one might find it rather confusing that WHO itself has another and slightly different definition for the term *E-Health*, which is the following: "the transfer of health resources and health care by electronic means. It encompasses three main areas:

- The delivery of health information, for health professionals and health consumers, through the Internet and telecommunications.
- Using the power of IT and e-commerce to improve public health services, e.g. through the education and training of health workers.
- The use of e-commerce and e-business practices in health systems management." [112]

Eysenbach [113], on the other hand, provided the following definition to *e-health* as a term and as a concept, and his definition remains to be broadly accepted till this date: "e-health is an emerging field in the intersection of medical informatics, public health and business, referring to health services and information delivered or enhanced through the Internet and related technologies. In a broader sense, the term characterizes not only a technical development, but also a state-of-mind, a way of thinking, an attitude, and a commitment for networked, global thinking, to improve health care locally, regionally, and worldwide by using information and communication technology." He also explained that the letter "e" in the term *eHealth* might refer to ten qualities, (1) efficiency, (2) enhancing quality of care, (3) evidence based, (4) empowerment of consumers and patients, (5) encouragement of a new relationship between the patient and health professional, (6) education of consumers and physicians through online sources, (7) enabling information exchange and communication in a standardized way between healthcare establishments, (8) extending the scope of healthcare beyond its conventional boundaries, (9) ethics, and (10) equity, so that everyone who needs *eHealth* would be able to receive it. For the context of our book, *eHealth* provides various monitoring services for older adults in need. For example, Cabrera-Umpiérrez et al. [66] described the developed functionalities of the *eHealth* services for European co-funded projects, which provided (a) personalized health monitoring, (b) health coaching, and (c) alerting and assisting services to assure the well-being of the older adult users during their daily activities. Our book is thus focused primarily on the *eHealth* services referring to the use cases (a) and (c) in that context.

Although much research has been carried out in the aforementioned fields that deal with older people monitoring at home in the recent years, several unsolved problems with existing tools persist, such as privacy issues [11, 64, 100], a lack of accuracy in detecting health-threatening problems [114], invasiveness [115] and intrusiveness [116, 117] of monitoring devices, and the fact that the monitoring systems are mostly meant for direct patient-physician communication, while physicians have a very limited time available per patient [16, 46, 118, 119]. Furthermore, the size and complexity of the available data from different electronic healthcare records is growing, which makes it harder for medical staff to analyze it and to make clinical decisions [120]. Thus, an automated detection of health-threatening situations and clinical decision support systems has become a new prerequisite for an effective home healthcare with limited manning [121].

1.2 Content and Audience of This Book

This book is intended for both geriatric care practitioners and engineers, who are developing or integrating monitoring solutions for older adults. On the one side, this book helps healthcare practitioners to familiarize with the available home monitoring technologies, and on the other side, it helps engineers to better understand the purposes and problems of monitoring older people at home through the insight into different scenarios and potential health-threatening situations and conditions of older adults with physical and/or mental impairments.

We start with reviewing a variety of well-known smart-home projects, which present an overview of the needed infrastructure and give an insight of what should be taken into consideration, when monitoring older people at home. The second chapter includes the summary of the existing notable reviews and the taxonomies of most common home monitoring scenarios. Subsequently, the third chapter reveals the spectrum of geriatric diseases and conditions mentioning the known approaches of solving them in home settings. Chapter 4 further reveals the available monitoring technology and possible automation of monitoring approaches, followed by examples of how to realize these solutions, what the pros and cons are, and what must be taken into consideration when implementing them in real home environments. The fifth chapter summarizes the available datasets, which are practically useful for developing health threat detection algorithms based on already monitored empirical data. Finally, in Chap. 6 we discuss some anticipated future challenges of applying monitoring technology for older adults and consequently propose possible measures and directions toward dealing with some common issues.

This book is based on numerous scientific articles, which were exclusively published in English, in a peer-reviewed text and were available as full works. Because of the rapid progression in technology and the relative lack of information in earlier years [24], our search was limited to articles in journals, book chapters, and conference proceedings written within the last 15 years, i.e., between 2001 and 2015; only few key relevant articles or book chapters with original sources from earlier years were included as exceptions. Additionally, several reports were cited to give more illustrative examples of approaches identified to be useful for monitoring geriatric patients at home, but which were not yet tested on older adults explicitly. As few exceptions, some web sites describing systems, devices, prototypes, and projects were included as references when the published literature did not offer adequate presentations of the projects. Searches using relevant keywords were conducted either in *Scopus*, *Elsevier*, *IEEE Xplore*, *Springer*, *PubMed*, and *PubMed Central* or using the *Google Scholar* search engine.

1.3 An Overview of the Relevant Smart-Home Projects

Table 1.1 summarizes several notable smart-home projects that are generally aimed at monitoring and assisting older people, including geriatric patients. The underlying aim of such projects was to explore the use of ambient and/or wearable sensing technology to monitor the well-being of older adults in their home environment.

The majority of the relevant smart-home projects are originating from Europe and America. For example, the well-known CASAS project, named for the Center for Advanced Studies in Adaptive Systems, at Washington State University (WSU) is active since 2007 and has established numerous smart-home test-beds equipped with sensors, which mainly aim to provide a noninvasive and unobtrusive assistive environment by monitoring ADL of the residents, including older patients [122–125]. The latest initiative of the CASAS project is to develop a "smart-home in a box" (SHiB), i.e., a small and portable home kit, lightweight in infrastructure, which can be implemented in a real home environment and extendable with minimal effort [123]. Noteworthy, the WSU CASAS database is the largest publicly available source of ADL datasets to date [126]. Meanwhile, researchers at the University of Missouri are using passive sensor networks installed in apartments of residents called as TigerPlace to detect changes in health status and offer clinical interventions helping the residents to age in place. The TigerPlace project aims to provide a long-term care model for seniors in terms of supportive health [9]. As another

Table 1.1 Smart-home projects with a perspective of monitoring geriatric patients

Reference	Coordinating research institution, country	Smart-home project	Datasets[a]	Type[b]
Cook et al. [123]	Washington State University, USA	CASAS, SHiB	✓, 65+, p	2, 4
Ranz et al. [9]	University of Missouri, Colombia	TigerPlace	✓, 65+, p	4
Stanford [119]	Oregon Health and Science University, USA	Elite Care	–, 65+, p	3
Abowd et al. [148]	Georgia Institute of Technology, USA	Aware Home	–	2 ~ 3
Kadouche et al. [131]	University of Sherbrooke, Canada	DOMUS	✓, s	2
Intille et al. [132]	Massachusetts Institute of Technology, USA	PlaceLab House_n	✓	3
Fleury et al. [134], Noury et al. [149]	TIMC-IMAG Laboratory of Grenoble, France	Health Smart Home, HIS^2	✓, s	2
Orpwood et al. [137]	Bath Institute of Medical Engineering, UK	Gloucester Smart House	–	2
S. Bjørneby et al. [138]	The Norwegian Centre for Dementia Research, Norway	ENABLE	–, 65+, p	4
Beul et al. [47]	Aachen University, Germany	Future Care Lab	–	1
Helal et al. [150]	University of Florida, USA	Gator Tech Smart House	✓, 65+, p	2
Yamazaki et al. [29, 142]	National Institute of Information and Communications Technology, Japan	Ubiquitous Home	✓, 65+, p	2
Tamura et al. [141]	Chiba University, Japan	Welfare Techno House	–, 65+, p	2
Kim et al. [144]	Pohang University of Science and Technology (POSTECH), South Korea	POSTECH's U-Health Smart Home	–	1
Chan et al. [136], Bonhomme et al. [102]	Laboratory for Analysis and Architecture of Systems (LAAS), France	PROSAFE, PROSAFE-extended	–, 65+, p	3
Callaghan et al. [151, 152]	University of Essex, UK	iDorm, iDorm2 (iSpace)	✓, s	3
Nishida et al. [143]	Electrotechnical Lab, Japan	SELF	–	1
Ivesen [153]	Danish Technological Institute (DTI), Denmark	DTI CareLab	–	1

(continued)

Table 1.1 (continued)

Reference	Coordinating research institution, country	Smart-home project	Datasets[a]	Type[b]
Sundar et al. [154]	University at Buffalo, USA	ActiveHome (X10)	–	4
Youngblood et al. [130]	The University of Texas at Arlington, USA	MavHome	–	1
Orcatech Technologies [155]	Oregon Center for Aging and Technology, USA	ORCATECH: Life Lab, Point of Care Lab	✓, 65+, p	2, 4
Coradeschi et al. [135], Palumbo et al. [156]	Örebro University, Sweden Real houses, and apartments in Italy, Spain, and Sweden	GiraffPlus	–, 65+, p	4
Soar et al. [147]	University of Southern Queensland, Australia	Queensland Smart Home Initiative (QSHI)	–, 65+, p	1, 4
Wilson et al. [145]	Australia's Commonwealth Scientific and Industrial Research Organization (CSIRO), Australia	Hospital Without Walls	–, 65+, p	2
Dodd et al. [146]	Australia's Commonwealth Scientific and Industrial Research Organization (CSIRO), Australia	Smarter Safer Home	–, 65+, p	4

[a]"Datasets" column indicates which smart-home projects have collected empirical datasets ("✓") and whether these projects include data from real older adults ("65+") and whether real medical patients were involved ("p"), or only simulated patients were used ("s"), i.e., healthy persons (often younger students) imitated symptoms of certain illnesses or alarming events, such as falls, or other behaviors of older patients.

[b]"Type" column classifies the test-beds of the reviewed smart-home projects into four main types, according to Tomita et al. [157]: 1 = "laboratory setting" (i.e., a facility at a research institution, which utilizes an infrastructure and sensory equipment that researchers find sufficient but is not meant for actual habitation), 2 = "prototype smart-home" (allows actual habitation, usually for a short-term, and is specifically designed for research purposes), 3 = "smart-home in use" (necessary infrastructure and monitoring technology is implemented in actual community settings, apartment complexes, or retirement housing units), 4 = "retrofitted smart-home" (i.e., a private home or an individual apartment is converted to a smart-home, by integrating (retrofitting) monitoring technology on top of existing home infrastructure).

example, Elite Care is an assisted living facility equipped with sensors to monitor indicators such as time in bed, body weight, and sleep restlessness using various sensors [119, 127]. The Aware Home project at Georgia Tech [128] employs a variety of sensors such as smart floor sensors, as well as assistive robots for monitoring and helping elderly. The MavHome [129, 130] at University of Texas at Arlington is another smart-home environment equipped with sensors, which records inhabitant interactions with many different devices, medicine-taking schedules, movement patterns, and vital signs. It aimed at providing healthcare assistance in living environments of older adults and people with disabilities. MavHome is one of the first projects, which proposed to apply machine learning approaches to create a smart-home that can act as an intelligent agent, i.e., which can adopt to its inhabitants, identify trends that could indicate health concerns or a need for transition to assisted care, or detect anomalies in regular living patterns that may require intervention. Other notable smart-home test-beds include DOMUS [131] at the University de Sherbrooke, and House_n project at the Massachusetts Institute of Technology [132]. Several smart-home projects in Europe include iDorm [133], Grenoble Health Smart Home [134], GiraffPlus [135], PROSAFE [136], Gloucester Smart House [137], ENABLE [138] for dementia patients, and Future Care Lab [47, 139]. The majority of these research projects monitor a subset of ADL tasks. There are also related joint initiatives such as the "Ambient Assisted Living Joint Programme" or "The Active and Assisted Living Joint Programme," supported by the European commission with the goal of enhancing the quality of life of older people across Europe through the use of AAL technologies and to support applied research on innovative ICT-enhanced services for aging well [44, 140]. As an example, in one of the most recent European projects, called as GiraffPlus [135], researchers develop and evaluate a complete system that collects daily behavioral and physiological data of older adults from distributed sensors; performs context recognition, a long-term trend analysis; and presents the information via a personalized interface. GiraffPlus supports social interaction between primary users (older citizens) and secondary users (formal and informal caregivers), thereby allowing caregivers to virtually visit an older person in the home.

Also in Asia, some notable smart-home projects were developed, such as the early "Welfare Techno Houses" across Japan [141], promoting independence for older and disabled persons and for improving their quality of life. For example, the large Takaoka Techno House [141] measured medical indicators such as electrocardiogram (ECG), body and excreta weights, and urinary volume, using sensor systems placed in the bed, toilet, and bathtub. The Ubiquitous Home project [29, 142] is another Japanese smart-home project, which applied passive infrared (PIR) sensors, cameras, microphones, pressure sensors, and radiofrequency identification (RFID) technology intended for monitoring living activities of residents, including older adults. The SELF smart-home project, also in Japan, monitored posture, body movement, breathing, and oxygen in the blood, using pressure sensor arrays, cameras, and microphones [143]. In South Korea, a POSTECH's U-Health smart-home project [144] is focused on establishing autonomic monitoring of home and its aging inhabitants in order to detect health problems, by applying different environmental wireless sensors and a wearable ECG monitor, and to provide assistance when needed.

In Oceania region, there are several noteworthy projects as well. For instance, the Hospital Without Walls project [145] is an early example of home telecare project in Australia that used a wireless wearable fall monitoring system based on small on-body sensors, which measured heart rate and body movements. The initial clinical scenario was monitoring older patients who were at risk of repeated falls. More recent projects include the Smarter Safer Home project [146] and the Queensland Smart Home Initiative (QSHI) [147]. The Smarter Safer Home platform [146] is aimed to enable aging Australians to live independently longer in their own homes. The primary goal of the proposed approach is to enhance the quality of life (QoL) for older patients and for the adult children supporting their aged parents. The aforementioned platform uses environmentally placed sensors for nonintrusive monitoring of human behaviors, extracting specific ADLs and predicting health decline or critical health situations from the changes in those ADLs. The Queensland Smart Home Initiative (QSHI) [147] program included so-called demonstrator smart-home, which involved feedback gathering from stakeholder visits, such as consumers, family members, care providers, and policy-makers, as well as 101 homes that are equipped with home telecare technologies and occupied by frail older adults or other people with special needs.

References

1. Christensen, K., Doblhammer, G., Rau, R., Vaupel, J.W.: Ageing populations: the challenges ahead. Lancet **374**(9696), 1196–1208 (2009)
2. European Commission: Demography Report 2010: Older, more numerous and diverse Europeans. Luxembourg (printed in Belgium) (2011)
3. Birkeland, A., Natvig, G.K.: Coping with ageing and failing health: a qualitative study among elderly living alone. Int. J. Nurs. Pract. **15**(4), 257–264 (2009)
4. Wrzus, C., Hänel, M., Wagner, J., Neyer, F.J.: Social network changes and life events across the life span: a meta-analysis. Psychol. Bull. **139**(1), 53–80 (2013)
5. Ke, S.R., Thuc, H., Lee, Y.J., Hwang, J.N., Yoo, J.H., Choi, K.H.: A review on video-based human activity recognition. Computers **2**(2), 88–131 (2013)
6. Popoola, O.P., Wang, K.: Video-based abnormal human behavior recognition: a review. IEEE Trans. Syst. Man Cybern. Part C Appl. Rev. **42**(6), 865–878 (2012)
7. Sabia, J.J.: There's no place like home: a hazard model analysis of aging in place among older homeowners in the PSID. Res. Aging **30**(1), 3–35 (2008)
8. Rantz, M., Skubic, M., Miller, S., Krampe, J.: Using technology to enhance aging in place. In: Helal, S., Mitra, S., Wong, J., Chang, C.K., Mokhtari, M. (eds.) Smart Homes and Health Telematics, pp. 169–176. Springer, Berlin/Heidelberg (2008)
9. Rantz, M.J., Skubic, M., Miller, S.J., Galambos, C., Alexander, G., Keller, J., Popescu, M.: Sensor technology to support aging in place. J. Am. Med. Dir. Assoc. **14**(6), 386–391 (2013)
10. Centers for Disease Control and Prevention: Healthy places terminology. http://www.cdc.gov/healthyplaces/terminology.htm (2009)
11. Steele, R., Lo, A., Secombe, C., Wong, Y.K.: Elderly persons' perception and acceptance of using wireless sensor networks to assist healthcare. Int. J. Med. Inf. **78**(12), 788–801 (2009)
12. Frits, T., Ana, L.-N., Francesca, C., Jérôme, M.: OECD Health Policy Studies Help Wanted? Providing and Paying for Long-Term Care: Providing and Paying for Long-Term Care. OECD, Paris (2011)
13. Hinck, S.: The lived experience of oldest-old rural adults. Qual. Health Res. **14**(6), 779–791 (2004)
14. Siddiqi, N., Clegg, A., Young, J.: Delirium in care homes. Rev. Clin. Gerontol. **19**(04), 309–316 (2009)
15. Tamura, T.: Home geriatric physiological measurements. Physiol. Meas. **33**(10), 47–65 (2012)
16. Alahmadi, A., Soh, B.: A smart approach towards a mobile e-health monitoring system architecture. In: 2011 International Conference on Research and Innovation in Information Systems (ICRIIS), pp. 1–5. Kuala Lumpur (2011)

17. Meystre, S.: The current state of telemonitoring: a comment on the literature. Telemed. E-Health **11**(1), 63–69 (2005)
18. Scanaill, C.N., Carew, S., Barralon, P., Noury, N., Lyons, D., Lyons, G.M.: A review of approaches to mobility telemonitoring of the elderly in their living environment. Ann. Biomed. Eng. **34**(4), 547–563 (2006)
19. Jiang, L., Liu, D., Yang, B.: Smart home research. In: Proceedings of 2004 International Conference on Machine Learning and Cybernetics, 2004, vol. 2, pp. 659–663. Shanghai (2004)
20. Morris, M.E., Adair, B., Miller, K., Ozanne, E., Hansen, R., Pearce, A.J., Santamaria, N., Viegas, L., Maureen, L., Said, C.M.: Smart-home technologies to assist older people to live well at home. J. Aging Sci. **1**(1), 1–9 (2013)
21. Ding, D., Cooper, R.A., Pasquina, P.F., Fici-Pasquina, L.: Sensor technology for smart homes. Maturitas **69**(2), 131–136 (2011)
22. Le, X.H.B., Di Mascolo, M., Gouin, A., Noury, N. Health smart home – towards an assistant tool for automatic assessment of the dependence of elders. In: 29th Annual International Conference of the IEEE Engineering in Medicine and Biology Society, 2007. EMBS 2007, pp. 3806–3809 (2007)
23. Grossi, F., Bianchi, V., Matrella, G., De Munari, I. Ciampolini, P.: An assistive home automation and monitoring system. In: International Conference on Consumer Electronics, 2008. ICCE 2008. Digest of technical papers, pp. 1–2. Las Vegas (2008)
24. Martin, S., Kelly, G., Kernohan, W.G., McCreight, B., Nugent, C.: Smart home technologies for health and social care support. In: Cochrane Database of Systematic Reviews. Wiley, Hoboken (2009)
25. Franchimon, F., Brink, M.: Matching technologies of home automation, robotics, assistance, geriatric telecare and telemedicine. Gerontechnology **8**(2) (2009)
26. Mann, W.C., Belchior, P., Tomita, M.R., Kemp, B.J.: Older adults' perception and use of PDAs, home automation system, and home health monitoring system. Top. Geriatr. Rehabil. **23**(1), 35–46 (2007)
27. Nourizadeh, S., Deroussent, C., Song, Y.-Q. Thomesse J.-P.: Medical and home automation sensor networks for senior citizens telehomecare. In: IEEE International Conference on Communications Workshops, pp. 1–5. Dresden (2009)
28. Pohl, P.D.K., Sikora, E.: Overview of the example domain: home automation. In: Software Product Line Engineering, pp. 39–52. Springer, Berlin/Heidelberg (2005)
29. Yamazaki, T.: The ubiquitous home. Int. J. Smart Home **1**(1), 17–22 (2007)
30. Wang, S., Ji, L., Li, A., Wu, J.: Body sensor networks for ubiquitous healthcare. J. Control Theory Appl. **9**(1), 3–9 (2011)
31. Sneha, S., Varshney, U.: Enabling ubiquitous patient monitoring: model, decision protocols, opportunities and challenges. Decis. Support Syst. **46**(3), 606–619 (2009)
32. Sampaio, D., Reis, L.P., Rodrigues, R.: A survey on ambient intelligence projects. In: 2012 7th Iberian Conference on Information Systems and Technologies (CISTI), pp. 1–6 (2012)
33. Rashidi, P., Mihailidis, A.: A survey on ambient-assisted living tools for older adults. IEEE J. Biomed. Health Inform. **17**(3), 579–590 (2013)
34. Sadri, F.: Ambient intelligence: a survey. ACM Comput. Surv. **43**(4), 36:1–36:66 (2011)
35. Cook, D.J., Augusto, J.C., Jakkula, V.R.: Ambient intelligence: technologies, applications, and opportunities. Pervasive Mob. Comput. **5**(4), 277–298 (2009)
36. Farella, E., O'Modhrain, S., Benini, L., Riccó, B.: Gesture signature for ambient intelligence applications: a feasibility study. In: Fishkin, K.P., Schiele, B., Nixon, P., Quigley, A. (eds.) Pervasive Computing, vol. 3968, pp. 288–304. Springer, Berlin/Heidelberg (2006)
37. Aztiria, A., Farhadi, G., Aghajan, H.: User behavior shift detection in intelligent environments. In: Bravo, J., Hervás, R., Rodríguez, M. (eds.) Ambient Assisted Living and Home Care, pp. 90–97. Springer, Berlin/Heidelberg (2012)
38. Miskelly, F.G.: Assistive technology in elderly care. Age Ageing **30**(6), 455–458 (2001)

39. Broekens, J., Heerink, M., Rosendal, H.: Assistive social robots in elderly care: a review. Gerontechnology **8**(2) (2009)
40. Megalingam, R.K., Radhakrishnan, V., Jacob, D.C., Unnikrishnan, D.K.M., Sudhakaran, A.K.: Assistive technology for elders: wireless intelligent healthcare gadget. In: 2011 IEEE Global Humanitarian Technology Conference (GHTC), pp. 296–300. Seattle (2011)
41. Chernbumroong, S., Cang, S., Atkins, A., Yu, H.: Elderly activities recognition and classification for applications in assisted living. Expert Syst. Appl. **40**(5), 1662–1674 (2013)
42. Vastenburg, M.H., Visser, T., Vermaas, M., Keyson, D.V.: Designing acceptable assisted living services for elderly users. In: Aarts, E., Crowley, J.L., de Ruyter, B., Gerhäuser, H., Pflaum, A., Schmidt, J., Wichert, R. (eds.) Ambient Intelligence, pp. 1–12. Springer, Berlin/Heidelberg (2008)
43. Graybill, E.M., McMeekin, P., Wildman, J.: Can aging in place be cost effective? a systematic review. PLoS One **9**(7), 102705 (2014)
44. European Commission: Ambient assisted living joint programme, DOI Httpwww Aal-Eur. EuprojectsAALCatalogueV3pdflast Checked 3011 2011 (2011)
45. Botia, J.A., Villa, A., Palma, J.: Ambient assisted living system for in-home monitoring of healthy independent elders. Expert Syst. Appl. **39**(9), 8136–8148 (2012)
46. Kanis, M., Alizadeh, S., Groen, J., Khalili, M., Robben, S., Bakkes, S., Kröse, B.: Ambient monitoring from an elderly-centred design perspective: what, who and how. In: Keyson, D.V., Maher, M.L., Streitz, N., Cheok, A., Augusto, J.C., Wichert, R., Englebienne, G., Aghajan, H., Kröse, B.J.A. (eds.) Ambient Intelligence, pp. 330–334. Springer, Berlin/Heidelberg (2011)
47. Beul, S., Klack, L., Kasugai, K., Moellering, C., Roecker, C., Wilkowska, W., Ziefle, M.: Between innovation and daily practice in the development of AAL systems: learning from the experience with today's systems. In: Szomszor, M., Kostkova, P. (eds.) Electronic Healthcare, pp. 111–118. Springer, Berlin/Heidelberg (2012)
48. Augusto, J.C., Huch, M., Kameas, A., Maitland, J., McCullagh, P.J., Roberts, J., Sixsmith, A., Wichert, R.: Handbook of Ambient Assisted Living: Technology for Healthcare, Rehabilitation and Well-Being. IOS Press, Washington, DC (2012)
49. Cardinaux, F., Bhowmik, D., Abhayaratne, C., Hawley, M.S.: Video based technology for ambient assisted living: a review of the literature. J. Ambient Intell. Smart Environ. **3**(3), 253–269 (2011)
50. Dang, S., Dimmick, S., Kelkar, G.: Evaluating the evidence base for the use of home telehealth remote monitoring in elderly with heart failure. Telemed. E-Health **15**(8), 783–796 (2009)
51. Ludwig, W., Wolf, K.-H., Duwenkamp, C., Gusew, N., Hellrung, N., Marschollek, M., Wagner, M., Haux, R.: Health-enabling technologies for the elderly – an overview of services based on a literature review. Comput. Methods Programs Biomed. **106**(2), 70–78 (2012)
52. Klose, H.-P., Braecklein, M., Nelles, S.: Telehealth – home-based self-monitoring of elderly chronically sick or at-risk patients. In: Dössel, O., Schlegel, W.C. (eds.) World Congress on Medical Physics and Biomedical Engineering, vol. 25/7, pp. 931–935. Springer, Berlin/Heidelberg (2009). 7–12 Sept 2009, Munich
53. Pieper, M., Stroetmann, K.: Chapter 9: Patients and EHRs tele home monitoring reference scenario. In: Stephanidis, C. (ed.) Universal Access in Health Telematics, pp. 77–87. Springer, Berlin/Heidelberg (2005)
54. Martín-Lesende, I., Orruño, E., Bilbao, A., Vergara, I., Cairo, M.C., Bayón, J.C., Reviriego, E., Romo, M.I., Larrañaga, J., Asua, J., Abad, R., Recalde, E.: Impact of telemonitoring home care patients with heart failure or chronic lung disease from primary care on healthcare resource use (the TELBIL study randomised controlled trial). BMC Health Serv. Res. **13**(1), 118 (2013)
55. Paré, G., Jaana, M., Sicotte, C.: Systematic review of home telemonitoring for chronic diseases: the evidence base. J. Am. Med. Inform. Assoc. **14**(3), 269–277 (2007)

56. Rehman, A., Mustafa, M., Javaid, N., Qasim, U., Khan, Z.A.: Analytical Survey of Wearable Sensors, arXiv:1208.2376 (2012)
57. González-Valenzuela, S., Chen, M., Leung, V.C.M.: Mobility support for health monitoring at home using wearable sensors. IEEE Trans. Inf. Technol. Biomed. **15**(4), 539–549 (2011)
58. Dagtas, S., Pekhteryev, G., Sahinoglu Z.: Multi-stage real time health monitoring via ZigBee in smart homes. In: 21st International Conference on Advanced Information Networking and Applications Workshops, 2007, AINAW '07, vol. 2, pp. 782–786 (2007)
59. Chi, Y.M., Deiss,S.R., Cauwenberghs, G.: Non-contact low power EEG/ECG electrode for high density wearable biopotential sensor networks. In: Sixth International Workshop on Wearable and Implantable Body Sensor Networks, 2009. BSN 2009, pp. 246–250 (2009)
60. Cheng, L., Shum, V., Kuntze, G., McPhillips, G.,Wilson, A., Hailes, S., Kerwin, D., Kerwin, G.: A wearable and flexible bracelet computer for on-body sensing. In: 2011 IEEE Consumer Communications and Networking Conference (CCNC), pp. 860–864 (2011)
61. Dishman, E.: Inventing wellness systems for aging in place. Computer **37**(5), 34–41 (2004)
62. Rodeschini, G.: Gerotechnology: a new kind of care for aging? an analysis of the relationship between older people and technology. Nurs. Health Sci. **13**(4), 521–528 (2011)
63. Bestente, G., Bazzani, M., Frisiello, A., Fiume, A., Mosso, D., Pernigotti, L.M.: DREAM: emergency monitoring system for the elderly. Gerontechnology **7**(2) (2008)
64. Wild, K., Boise, L., Lundell, J., Foucek, A.: Unobtrusive in-home monitoring of cognitive and physical health: reactions and perceptions of older adults. J. Appl. Gerontol. **27**(2), 181–200 (2008)
65. World Health Organisation: WHO/eHealth. http://www.who.int/topics/ehealth/en/ (2015). Accessed 16 Sept 2015
66. Cabrera-Umpiérrez, M.F., Jiménez, V., Fernández, M.M., Salazar, J., Huerta, M.A.: eHealth services for the elderly at home and on the move. In: IST-Africa 2010, pp. 1–6. Durban (2010)
67. Institute of Medicine (US) Committee on Evaluating Clinical Applications of Telemedicine: Telemedicine: A Guide to Assessing Telecommunications in Health Care. National Academies Press, Washington, DC (1996)
68. Chaudhry, S.I., Mattera, J.A., Curtis, J.P., Spertus, J.A., Herrin, J., Lin, Z., Phillips, C.O., Hodshon, B.V., Cooper, L.S., Krumholz, H.M.: Telemonitoring in patients with heart failure. N. Engl. J. Med. **363**(24), 2301–2309 (2010)
69. Le, X.H.B., Di Mascolo, M., Gouin, A., Noury, N.: Health smart home for elders – a tool for automatic recognition of activities of daily living. In: 30th Annual International Conference of the IEEE Engineering in Medicine and Biology Society, 2008. EMBS 2008, pp. 3316–3319 (2008)
70. Choukeir, A., Fneish, B., Zaarour, N., Fahs, W., Ayache, M.: Health smart home. Int. Comput. Sci. Issues **7**(6), 126–130 (2010)
71. Rialle, V., Duchene, F., Noury, N., Bajolle, L., Demongeot, J.: Health 'smart' home: information technology for patients at home. Telemed. J. E Health **8**(4), 395–409 (2002)
72. O'Donoghue, J., Wichert, R., Divitini, M.: Introduction to the thematic issue: home-based health and wellness measurement and monitoring. J. Ambient Intell. Smart Environ. **4**(5), 399–401 (2012)
73. Vasilakos, A., Pedrycz, W.: Ambient Intelligence, Wireless Networking, and Ubiquitous Computing. Artech House, Boston (2006)
74. Crutzen, C.K.M.: Invisibility and the meaning of ambient intelligence. Int. Rev. Inf. Ethics **6**, 52–62 (2006)
75. Fausset, C.B., Kelly, A.J., Rogers, W.A., Fisk, A.D.: Challenges to aging in place: understanding home maintenance difficulties. J. Hous. Elder. **25**(2), 125–141 (2011)
76. Innotraction Solutions Inc: Continuing Care Health Technologies Roadmap: Aging in the Right Place. Alberta Advanced Education and Technology, Calgary (2009)
77. Fozard, J.L., Rietsema, J., Herman, B., Graafmans, J.A.M.: Gerontechnology: creating enabling environments for the challenges and opportunities of aging. Educ. Gerontol. **26**(4), 331–344 (2000)

78. Seelman, K.D., Palmer, C.V., Ortmann, A., Mormer, E., Guthrie, O., Miele, J., Brabyn, J.: Quality-of-life technology for vision and hearing loss [Highlights of recent developments and current challenges in technology]. IEEE Eng. Med. Biol. Mag. **27**(2), 40–55 (2008)
79. Stowe, S., Hopes, J., Mulley, G.: Gerotechnology series: 2. Walking aids. Eur. Geriatr. Med. **1**(2), 122–127 (2010)
80. Harman, D., Craigie, S.: Gerotechnology series: toileting aids. Eur. Geriatr. Med. **2**(5), 314–318 (2011)
81. Burdick, D., Kwon, S.: Gerotechnology: Research and Practice in Technology and Aging. Springer, New York (2004)
82. Cook, A.M., Polgar, J.M.: Assistive Technologies: Principles and Practice. Elsevier Health Sciences, Philadelphia (2014)
83. Lushai, G., Cox, T.: Assisted Living Technology: A Market and Technology Review. Life Sciences-Healthcare and the Institute of Bio-Sensing Technology, Bristol (2012)
84. Lewin, D., Adshead, S., Glennon, B., Williamson, B., Moore, T., Damodaran, L., Hansell, P.: Assisted Living Technologies for Older and Disabled People in 2030. Plum Consulting, London (2010)
85. Kalra, L., Zhao, X., Soto, A.J., Milios, E.: Detection of daily living activities using a two-stage Markov model. J. Ambient Intell. Smart Environ. **5**(3), 273–285 (2013)
86. Bosse, T., Hoogendoorn, M., Klein, M.C.A., Treur, J.: An ambient agent model for monitoring and analysing dynamics of complex human behaviour. J. Ambient Intell. Smart Environ. **3**(4), 283–303 (2011)
87. Franco, G.C., Gallay, F., Berenguer, M., Mourrain, C., Couturier, P.: Non-invasive monitoring of the activities of daily living of elderly people at home – a pilot study of the usage of domestic appliances. J. Telemed. Telecare **14**(5), 231–235 (2008)
88. Sun, Y.: Design of low cost human ADL signal acquire system based on wireless wearable MEMS sensor. In: Jin, D., Lin, S. (eds.) Advances in Computer Science, Intelligent System and Environment, vol. 104, pp. 703–707. Springer, Berlin/Heidelberg (2011)
89. Chang, C.-H., Lai, Y.-L., Chen, C.-C.: Implement the RFID position based system of automatic tablets packaging machine for patient safety. J. Med. Syst. **36**(6), 3463–3471 (2012)
90. Dobkin, B.H., Dorsch, A.: The promise of mHealth daily activity monitoring and outcome assessments by wearable sensors. Neurorehabil. Neural Repair **25**(9), 788–798 (2011)
91. Luštrek, M., Kaluža, B.: Fall detection and activity recognition with machine learning. Informatica **33**, 205–212 (2009)
92. Pogorelc, B., Gams, M.: Discovering the chances of health problems and falls in the elderly using data mining. In: Ohsawa, Y., Abe, A. (eds.) Advances in Chance Discovery, pp. 163–175. Springer, Berlin/Heidelberg (2013)
93. Yu, M., Rhuma, A., Naqvi, S.M., Wang, L., Chambers, J.: A posture recognition-based fall detection system for monitoring an elderly person in a smart home environment. Ieee Trans. Inf. Technol. Biomed. **16**(6), 1274–1286 (2012)
94. Uslu, G., Altun, O., Baydere, S.: A Bayesian approach for indoor human activity monitoring. In: 2011 11th International Conference on Hybrid Intelligent Systems (HIS), pp. 324–327. Malacca (2011)
95. Suryadevara, N.K., Gaddam, A., Rayudu, R.K., Mukhopadhyay, S.C.: Wireless sensors network based safe home to care elderly people: behaviour detection. Sens. Actuators Phys. **186**, 277–283 (2012)
96. Arcelus, A., Holtzman, M., Goubran, R., Sveistrup, H., Guitard, P., Knoefel, F.: Analysis of commode grab bar usage for the monitoring of older adults in the smart home environment. Conference Proceedings Annual International Conference of the IEEE Engineering in Medicine and Biology Society, vol. 2009, pp. 6155–6158. Minneapolis (2009)
97. Przybelski, R.J., Shea, T.A.: Falls in the geriatric patient. WMJ Off. Publ. State Med. Soc. Wis. **100**(2), 53–56 (2001)
98. Moyer, V.A., U.S. Preventive Services Task Force: Prevention of falls in community-dwelling older adults: U.S. Preventive Services Task Force recommendation statement. Ann. Intern. Med. **157**(3), 197–204 (2012)
99. Aggarwal, J.K., Ryoo, M.S.: Human activity analysis: a review. ACM Comput. Surv. **43**(3), 16:1–16:43 (2011)

100. Bharucha, A.J., London, A.J., Barnard, D., Wactlar, H., Dew, M.A., Reynolds 3rd C.F.: Ethical considerations in the conduct of electronic surveillance research. J. Law Med. Ethics J. Am. Soc. Law Med. Ethics **34**(3), 611–619, 482 (2006)
101. Chen, M.-Y., Hauptmann, A., Bharucha, A., Wactlar, H., Yang, Y.: Human activity analysis for geriatric care in nursing homes. In: The Era of Interactive Media, pp. 53–61. Springer, New York (2013)
102. Bonhomme, S., Campo, E., Esteve, D., Guennec, J.: An extended PROSAFE platform for elderly monitoring at home. Conf. Proc. Annu. Int. Conf. IEEE Eng. Med. Biol. Soc. IEEE Eng. Med. Biol. Soc. Conf. **2007**, 4056–4059 (2007)
103. Corchado, J.M., Bajo, J., Tapia, D.I., Abraham, A.: Using heterogeneous wireless sensor networks in a telemonitoring system for healthcare. IEEE Trans. Inf. Technol. Biomed. **14**(2), 234–240 (2010)
104. Hägglund, M., Scandurra, I., Koch, S.: Scenarios to capture work processes in shared homecare – from analysis to application. Int. J. Med. Inf. **79**(6), e126–e134 (2010)
105. Liuqing, Y.: Video monitoring communication system design based on wireless mesh networks. In: 2012 International Conference on Computer Science and Electronics Engineering (ICCSEE), vol. 3, pp. 503–507. Hangzhou (2012)
106. Kim, H., Jarochowski, B., Ryu, D.: A proposal for a home-based health monitoring system for the elderly or disabled. In: Miesenberger, K., Klaus, J., Zagler, W., Karshmer, A. (eds.) Computers Helping People with Special Needs, Proceedings of 10th International Conference on Computers Helping People with Special Needs (ICCHP) 2006, (LNCS), vol. 4061, pp. 473–479. Springer, Berlin (2006)
107. Snogdal, L.S., Folkestad, L., Elsborg, R., Remvig, L.S., Beck-Nielsen, H., Thorsteinsson, B., Jennum, P., Gjerstad, M., Juhl, C.B.: Detection of hypoglycemia associated EEG changes during sleep in type 1 diabetes mellitus. Diabetes Res. Clin. Pract. **98**(1), 91–97 (2012)
108. Kozlovszky, M., Sicz-Mesziár, J., Ferenczi, J., Márton, J., Windisch, G., Kozlovszky, V., Kotcauer, P., Boruzs, A., Bogdanov, P., Meixner, Z., Karóczkai, K.: Combined health monitoring and emergency management through android based mobile device for elderly people. In: Nikita, K.S., Lin, J.C., Fotiadis, D.I., Arredondo Waldmeyer, M.-T. (eds.) Wireless Mobile Communication and Healthcare. S. Ács, vol. 83, pp. 268–274. Springer, Berlin/Heidelberg (2012)
109. Huang, Y.-C., Lu, C.-H., Yang, T.-H., Fu, L.-C., Wang, C.-Y.: Context-aware personal diet suggestion system. In: Lee, Y., Bien, Z.Z., Mokhtari, M., Kim, J.T., Park, M., Kim, J., Lee, H., Khalil, I. (eds.) Aging Friendly Technology for Health and Independence, pp. 76–84. Springer, Berlin/Heidelberg (2010)
110. Pagliari, C., Sloan, D., Gregor, P., Sullivan, F., Detmer, D., Kahan, J.P., Oortwijn, W., MacGillivray, S.: What is eHealth (4): a scoping exercise to map the field. J. Med. Internet Res. **7**(1), e9 (2005)
111. U.S. National Library of Medicine: MeSH browser – 2015. Medical Subject Headings. https://www.nlm.nih.gov/mesh/MBrowser.html (2015). Accessed 16 Sept 2015
112. World Health Organisation: WHO/E-Health. http://www.who.int/trade/glossary/story021/en/ (2015). Accessed 16 Sept 2015
113. Eysenbach, G.: What is e-health? J. Med. Internet Res. **3**(2), e20 (2001)
114. Zhang, Y.: Real-time development of patient-specific alarm algorithms for critical care. In: 29th Annual International Conference of the IEEE Engineering in Medicine and Biology Society, 2007. EMBS 2007, pp. 4351–4354. Lyon (2007)
115. Watson, S., Wenzel, R.R., di Matteo, C., Meier, B., Lüscher, T.F.: Accuracy of a new wrist cuff oscillometric blood pressure device comparisons with intraarterial and mercury manometer measurements. Am. J. Hypertens. **11**(12), 1469–1474 (1998)
116. Lin, Y.: A natural contact sensor paradigm for nonintrusive and real-time sensing of biosignals in human-machine interactions. IEEE Sens. J. **11**(3), 522–529 (2011)
117. Mann, W.C., Marchant, T., Tomita, M., Fraas, L., Stanton, K.: Elder acceptance of health monitoring devices in the home. Care Manag. J. J. Case Manag. J. Long Term Home Health Care **3**(2), 91–98 (2001/2002)

118. Mapundu, Z., Simonnet, T., van der Walt, J.S.: A videoconferencing tool acting as a home-based healthcare monitoring robot for elderly patients. Stud. Health Technol. Inform. **182**, 180–188 (2012)
119. Stanford, V.: Using pervasive computing to deliver elder care. IEEE Pervasive Comput. **1**(1), 10–13 (2002)
120. WHO: WHO/Knowledge translation framework for ageing and health. http://www.who.int/ageing/publications/knowledge_translation/en/index.html. Accessed 22 Nov 2012
121. Eskola, M.J., Nikus, K.C., Voipio-Pulkki, L.-M., Huhtala, H., Parviainen, T., Lund, J., Ilva, T., Porela, P.: Comparative accuracy of manual versus computerized electrocardiographic measurement of J-, ST- and T-wave deviations in patients with acute coronary syndrome. Am. J. Cardiol. **96**(11), 1584–1588 (2005)
122. Crandall, A.S., Cook, D.J.: Smart home in a box: a large scale smart home deployment. In: Workshop Proceedings of the 8th International Conference on Intelligent Environments, Guanajuato, 26–29 June 2012, vol. 13, pp. 169–178 (2012)
123. Cook, D.J., Crandall, A.S., Thomas, B.L., Krishnan, N.C.: CASAS: a smart home in a box. Computer **46**(7), 62–69 (2013)
124. Cook, D., Schmitter-Edgecombe, M., Crandall, A., Sanders, C., Thomas, B.: Collecting and disseminating smart home sensor data in the CASAS project. In: Proceedings of CHI09 Workshop on Developing Shared Home Behavior Datasets to Advance HCI and Ubiquitous Computing Research. Boston (2009)
125. Rashidi, P., Cook, D.J.: Keeping the resident in the loop: adapting the smart home to the user. IEEE Trans. Syst. Man Cybern. Part Syst. Hum. **39**(5), 949–959 (2009)
126. Cook, D., Crandall, A., Ghasemzadeh, H., Holder, L., Schmitter-Edgecombe, M., Shirazi, B., Taylor, M.: WSU CASAS Datasets. WSU CASAS. http://ailab.wsu.edu/casas/datasets/ (2012). Accessed 1 Oct 2013
127. Home/Elite Care/Senior Living Tigard, Milwaukie, Vancouver.: Elite Care. http://www.elitecare.com/. Accessed 23 Aug 2013
128. Essa, I.A.: Aware Home: Sensing, Interpretation, and Recognition of Everday Activities. https://smartech.gatech.edu/handle/1853/11279 (2005). Accessed 23 Aug 2013
129. Das, S.K., Cook, D.J.: Health monitoring in an agent-based smart home. In: Proceedings of the International Conference on Smart Homes and Health Telematics (ICOST), pp. 3–14. Singapore (2004)
130. Youngblood, G.M., Holder, L.B., Cook, D.J.: Managing adaptive versatile environments. In: Third IEEE International Conference on Pervasive Computing and Communications, 2005. PerCom 2005, pp. 351–360 (2005)
131. Kadouche, R., Pigot, H., Abdulrazak, B., Giroux, S.: User's behavior classification model for smart houses occupant prediction. In: Chen, L., Nugent, C.D., Biswas, J., Hoey, J. (eds.) Activity Recognition in Pervasive Intelligent Environments, pp. 149–164. Atlantis Press, Paris (2011)
132. Intille, S.S., Larson, K., Tapia, E.M., Beaudin, J.S., Kaushik, P., Nawyn, J., Rockinson, R.: Using a live-in laboratory for ubiquitous computing research. In: Fishkin, K.P., Schiele, B., Nixon, P., Quigley, A. (eds.) Pervasive Computing, pp. 349–365. Springer, Berlin/Heidelberg (2006)
133. Duman, H., Hagras, H., Callaghan, V.: Adding intelligence to ubiquitous computing environments. In: Lee, P.R.S.T., Loia, P.V. (eds.) Computational Intelligence for Agent-Based Systems, pp. 61–102. Springer, Berlin/Heidelberg (2007)
134. Fleury, A., Noury, N., Vacher, M., Glasson, H., Seri, J.F.: Sound and speech detection and classification in a health smart home. Conference Proceedings Annual International Conference of the IEEE Engineering in Medicine and Biology Society, vol. 2008, pp. 4644–4647. Vancouver (2008)
135. Coradeschi, S., Cesta, A., Cortellessa, G., Coraci, L., Galindo, C., Gonzalez, J., Karlsson, L., Forsberg, A., Frennert, S., Furfari, F., Loutfi, A., Orlandini, A., Palumbo, F., Pecora, F., von Rump, S., Štimec, A., Ullberg, J., Ötslund, B.: GiraffPlus: a system for monitoring activities and physiological parameters and promoting social interaction for elderly. In: Hippe, Z.S., Kulikowski, J.L., Mroczek, T., Wtorek, J. (eds.) Human-Computer Systems Interaction:

Backgrounds and Applications, vol. 3, pp. 261–271. Springer International Publishing, New York (2014)
136. Chan, M., Campo, E., Esteve, D.: PROSAFE, a multisensory remote monitoring system for the elderly or the handicapped. Indep. Living Pers. Disabil. Elder. People, 89–95 (2003)
137. Orpwood, R., Gibbs, C., Adlam, T., Faulkner, R., Meegahawatte, D.: The gloucester smart house for people with dementia – user-interface aspects. In: Keates, S., Clarkson, J., Langdon, P., Robinson, P. (eds.) Designing a More Inclusive World, pp. 237–245. Springer, London (2004)
138. Bjørneby, S., Topo, P., Cahill, S., Begley, E., Jones, K., Hagen, I., Macijauskiene, J., Holthe, T.: Ethical considerations in the ENABLE project. Dementia **3**(3), 297–312 (2004)
139. Klack, L., Möllering, C., Ziefle, M., Schmitz-Rode, T.: Future care floor: a sensitive floor for movement monitoring and fall detection in home environments. In: Lin, J.C., Nikita, K.S. (eds.) Wireless Mobile Communication and Healthcare, pp. 211–218. Springer, Berlin/Heidelberg (2011)
140. The Active and Assisted Living Joint Programme (AAL JP): Digital Agenda for Europe. ec.europa.eu//digital-agenda/en/active-and-assisted-living-joint-programme-aal-jp. Accessed 2 Oct 2014
141. Tamura, T., Kawarada, A., Nambu, M., Tsukada, A., Sasaki, K., Yamakoshi, K.-I.: E-healthcare at an experimental welfare techno house in Japan. Open Med. Inform. J. **1**, 1–7 (2007)
142. Yamazaki, T.: Ubiquitous home: real-life testbed for home context-aware service. In: First International Conference on Testbeds and Research Infrastructures for the Development of Networks and Communities, 2005. Tridentcom 2005, pp. 54–59. Trento (2005)
143. Nishida, Y., Hori, T., Suehiro, T., Hirai, S.: Sensorized environment for self-communication based on observation of daily human behavior. In: 2000 IEEE/RSJ International Conference on Intelligent Robots and Systems, 2000. (IROS 2000). Proceedings, vol. 2, pp. 1364–1372. Takamatsu (2000)
144. Kim, J., Choi, H., Wang, H., Agoulmine, N., Deerv, M.J., Hong, J.W.-K.: POSTECH's u-health smart home for elderly monitoring and support. In: 2010 IEEE International Symposium on a World of Wireless Mobile and Multimedia Networks (WoWMoM), pp. 1–6. Montreal (2010)
145. Wilson, L.S., Gill, R.W., Sharp, I.F., Joseph, J., Heitmann, S.A., Chen, C.F., Dadd, M.J., Kajan, A., Collings, A.F., Gunaratnam, M.: Building the hospital without walls – a CSIRO home telecare initiative. Telemed. J. Off. J. Am. Telemed. Assoc. **6**(2), 275–281 (2000)
146. Zhang, Q., Karunanithi, M., Rana, R., Liu, J.: Determination of activities of daily living of independent living older people using environmentally placed sensors. Conference Proceedings Annual International Conference of the IEEE Engineering in Medicine and Biology Society, vol. 2013, pp. 7044–7047. Osaka (2013)
147. Soar, J., Livingstone, A., Wang, S.-Y.: A case study of an ambient living and wellness management health care model in Australia. In: Mokhtari, M., Khalil, I., Bauchet, J., Zhang, D., Nugent, C. (eds.) Ambient Assistive Health and Wellness Management in the Heart of the City, pp. 48–56. Springer, Berlin/Heidelberg (2009)
148. Abowd, G.D., Mynatt, E.D.: Designing for the human experience in smart environments. In: Cook, D.J., Das, S.K. (eds.) Smart Environments, pp. 151–174. Wiley, Hoboken (2005)
149. Noury, N., Virone, G., Creuzet, T.: The health integrated smart home information system (HIS2): rules based system for the localization of a human. In: 2nd Annual International IEEE-EMB Special Topic Conference on Microtechnologies in Medicine and Biology, pp. 318–321 (2002)
150. Helal, S., Mann, W., El-Zabadani, H., King, J., Kaddoura, Y., Jansen, E.: The gator tech smart house: a programmable pervasive space. Computer **38**(3), 50–60 (2005)
151. Callaghan, V., Colley, M., Hagras, H., Chin, J., Doctor, F., Clarke, G.: Programming iSpaces – a tale of two paradigms. In: Steventon, A., Wright, S. (eds.) Intelligent Spaces, pp. 389–421. Springer, London (2006)

152. Intelligent Inhabited Environments Group: iSpace. Intelligent Inhabited Environments Group, Department of Computer Science, University of Essex, United Kingdom. http://cswww.essex.ac.uk/Research/iieg/idorm2/index.htm (2010). Accessed 8 Aug 2014
153. Iversen, J.: CareLab. Try More Than 15 New Welfare Technologies. http://www.dti.dk/try-more-than-15-new-welfare-technologies/34367?cms.query=carelab (2014). Accessed 12 Sept 2014
154. Machiko, W.C.M., Tomita, R.: Use of currently available smart home technology by frail elders: process and outcomes. Top. Geriatr. Rehabil. **23**(1), 24–34 (2006)
155. OHSU: ORCATECH Technologies. Oregon Health & Science University. http://www.ohsu.edu/xd/research/centers-institutes/orcatech/tech/index.cfm (2014). Accessed 6 Sept 2014
156. Palumbo, F., Ullberg, J., Štimec, A., Furfari, F., Karlsson, L., Coradeschi, S.: Sensor network infrastructure for a home care monitoring system. Sensors **14**(3), 3833–3860 (2014)
157. Tomita, M., Russ, L.S., Sridhar, R., Naughton M, B.J.: Smart home with healthcare technologies for community-dwelling older adults. In: Al-Qutayri, M.A. (ed.) Smart Home Systems. InTech. Rijeka (2010)

Chapter 2
Reviews and Taxonomies

Abstract This chapter summarizes the existing review articles in the field of monitoring and diagnosing older adults at risk of health deterioration, in the context of smart-homes. We provide taxonomy of these notable review articles, characterizing their aims and reviewing approaches of proposed monitoring systems capable of detecting health threats in smart-home settings. We included reviews, which focus on describing technology, applications, costs, and quality of monitoring services. These reviews greatly help to orientate in the assortment of available monitoring solutions for various scenarios.

Keywords Patient monitoring systems • Smart-home projects • Review • Technology • Application • Cost • Quality of service (QoS) • Ambient assisted living (AAL) • Taxonomy

Over the past decade, the number of publications concerning the field of monitoring older adults at home has grown significantly. To structure an overview of the individual review articles, including their purpose and approaches, a taxonomy may be defined to arrange them into various groups having similar characteristics.

Various categories may be used for a taxonomy to distinguish between different approaches (e.g., in random order): patient-centric versus physician-centric approaches, vision-based versus non-vision-based systems, active versus passive sensing, mobile versus stationary sensors, various scenario assumptions (health condition and disabilities, single patient vs. multiple patients, number of rooms at home, etc.), cost, number of monitored parameters, sensor modality, long-term monitoring versus short-term monitoring, nonintrusive versus holistic intrusive methods, etc. The various review works that are discussed in the next chapter have used different taxonomies.

J. Klonovs et al., *Distributed Computing and Monitoring Technologies for Older Patients*, SpringerBriefs in Computer Science,
DOI 10.1007/978-3-319-27024-1_2

2.1 Previous Reviews

A number of comprehensive reviews were written which summarized the important proposals of monitoring and diagnosing at home older adults at risk of health deterioration, in the context of smart-homes, the last one being published in March 2015. All reviews discuss both vision and non-vision-based monitoring technology. Some of these reviews explicitly mentioned medical application contexts [1–13], and some did not [14]. These reviews can be classified into different overlapping groups according to the viewpoints used during the review process. The viewpoints are (a) technology centric, (b) application centric, (c) cost centric, and (d) quality of service (QoS) centric. Figure 2.1 illustrates these four groups and corresponding reviews from the literature. Technology-centric reviews included discussions and summarized methods regarding core technologies, such as object segmentation, feature extraction, activity detection and recognition, clinically important symptom detection, etc. Application-centric reviews discussed and summarized methods related to applications such as fall detection, detection of ADL, detection of instrumental activities, detection of sick samples for diagnosis, etc. Cost-centric reviews discussed the expenditures required for implementation of activity monitoring systems. The QoS-centric reviews discussed and summarized the service quality of the methods in the area of activity monitoring and elderly assisted smart-homes. Service quality can be defined in terms of validation study, performance, user adaptability, sensitivity, etc., which is usually assessed based on the outcomes. Service quality naturally is focused on benefitting an end user (an older adult), and when this end user is a patient, QoS-centric reviews often discuss patient centeredness of the reviewed approaches. They often tend to summarize outcomes of different telemonitoring solutions and to give best practice recommendations for improving quality of service for older adults.

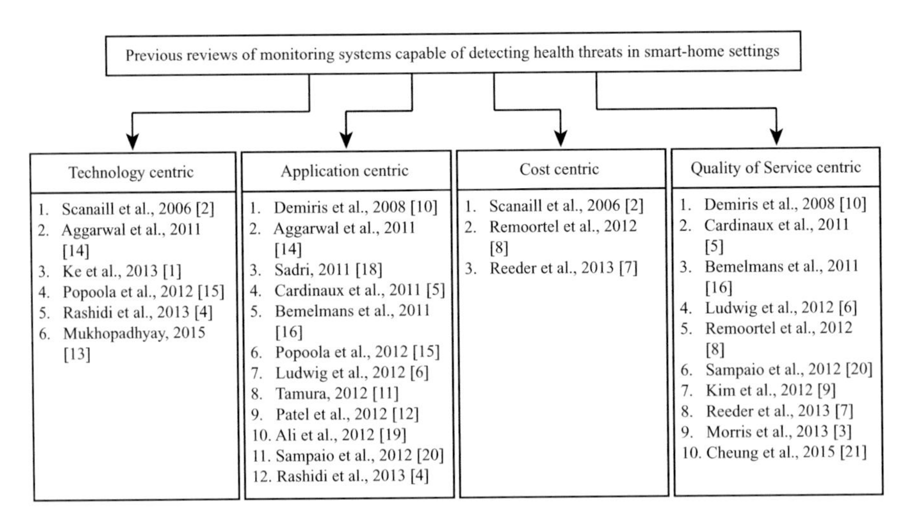

Fig. 2.1 Categories of existing reviews in the literature in terms of their viewpoints (mentioning the first author and year of publication for each reference)

Among the previous reviews, technology- and application-centric reviews achieved good consideration in the study of automated monitoring and diagnosis in smart-homes. Though technology-centric reviews in the literature thoroughly addressed the core technologies used in this area (e.g., describing system architecture, integrated sensors, proposed algorithms, communication protocols, etc.), application-centric reviews focus on particular application area and may, for example, merely consider some subgroups of ADL, or instrumental activities, or generalized human activities in both medical and nonmedical contexts [1, 4, 5, 7]. Most of these application-centric reviews did not include comprehensively the issues of older patients in an assisted living environment; however, they have mentioned general scenarios of monitoring older adults at home. There is a very limited discussion of patient centeredness among these reviews, which only includes some discussions and summaries of the methods in terms of patient's necessity, services, and measuring parameters, such as handling adverse condition, assessing state of health, and in-home diagnosis methods. Moreover, the previous reviews did not discuss the methods for in-home diagnosis of patients and include less discussion regarding collection of datasets in the patient-centered contexts. Thus, in this book we systematically summarize the methods that came up as solutions by utilizing monitored data to the issues related to patient's necessity, services, and measuring diagnostic parameters of older adults in smart-home scenarios.

Table 2.1 further summarizes the main features and contents of these key review works in the domain of monitoring technologies and health threat detection in older adults, where the column *Topic* presents the reviews' context such as the algorithms for activity recognition, hardware tools available for monitoring, hospitality services available at home, and/or evaluation methods for monitoring systems. The column *Contents* presents the summaries of reviews, *Types of Analysis* notes the types of data (either quantitative or qualitative) used in the review in order to assess the existing literature and the application types (medical or general) considered in the reviews, and *Sensors Discussed* presents the types of sensors discussed in the reviews. The medical application in column 4 was drawn from the setup related to the medically ill patients, whereas the nonmedical or general application context was drawn from the setup not necessarily related to real patients or geriatrics. However, in Table 2.1 we have included reviews covering nonmedical applications, because the contents of the reviews included the literatures and the underlying objectives of monitoring activities and measuring physiological parameters of geriatric patients at home. In column 5, vision-based sensors include, for example, thermal cameras, RGB cameras, and/or infrared cameras. On the other hand, the most common non-vision-based sensors are microphones, accelerometers, heat sensors, flow sensors, pressure sensors, electromagnetic sensors, ultrasonic sensors, and particle sensors.

A notable study by Morris et al. [3] systematically reviewed smart-home technologies that assisted older adults to live well at home. This review is mainly quality of service (QoS) centric, because the authors only reviewed works, which assessed smart-home technologies in terms of effectiveness, feasibility, acceptability, and perceptions of older people. They indicated that only one study assessed effectiveness

Table 2.1 Summary of the review works in the fields of vision-based and non-vision-based patient monitoring and health threat detection technologies

References (first author and year of publication)	Topic	Contents/main contributions	Type of the analysis	Sensors discussed	Viewpoints covered	Number of citations (reviewed works)
J.K. Aggarwal, 2011 [14]	Human activity analysis	Taxonomy of human activity in terms of automated recognition complexity, tools for recognition, summarizing the services of different proposed methods, discussion about dataset creation and availability	Both qualitative and quantitative in nonmedical applications	Vision based	Technology and application centric	102
S.R. Ke, 2013 [1]	Tools for activity recognition	Discussing object detection methods, feature extraction and representation methods, machine learning methods, some example of activity recognition systems	Qualitative in both medical and nonmedical applications	Vision based	Technology centric	145
O.P. Popoola, 2012 [15]	Video analysis for abnormal human behavior detection	Summarizing the focus of previous review articles for behavior recognition, organizing the references for common tools and paradigms used, theme-based classification of previous research, listing of datasets	Qualitative in medical and surveillance applications	Vision based	Technology and application centric	141

C.N. Scanaill, 2006 [2]	Sensors used for mobility telemonitoring of elderly	Estimating expenditure for assisted independent aging, summarizing the characteristics of sensors, and corresponding pros and cons	Qualitative in medical applications	Vision and non-vision based	Technology and cost centric	59
F. Cardinaux, 2011 [5]	Video analysis for ambient assisted living	Application-centric listing of existing methods, services of existing methods for action detection, visual processing, and privacy of visual data	Qualitative in medical applications	Vision based	Application and QoS centric	72
G. Demiris, 2008 [10]	Systematic review of smart-home applications for aging society	Discussing technologies and models used in existing smart-home projects, categorizing them in accordance to monitoring of physiological, functional outcomes, safety and security, social interactions, emergency detection, and cognitive and sensory assistance	Qualitative in medical applications	Vision and non-vision based	Application and QoS centric	31 (114)

(continued)

Table 2.1 (continued)

References (first author and year of publication)	Topic	Contents/main contributions	Type of the analysis	Sensors discussed	Viewpoints covered	Number of citations (reviewed works)
B. Reeder, 2013 [7]	Health smart-homes and home-based consumer health technologies for independent aging	Classifying technologies into emerging, promising, and effective groups, summarizing the contribution of each article instead of subdivision of methods used, analyzing the study of environment for each article	Qualitative in medical applications	Vision and non-vision based	QoS centric	83 (31 key articles out of 1685 articles)
W. Ludwig, 2012 [6]	Services from health-enabling technologies	Handling adverse conditions such as fall detection and cardiac emergencies, assessing state of health such as recognition of diseases and medical conditions, consultation and education for the use of services, motivation and feedback from the user, service ordering, social inclusion of telehealth services	Qualitative in medical applications	Vision and non-vision based	Application and QoS centric	47 (27 key articles out of 1447 articles)
H.V. Remoortel, 2012 [8]	Validity study of activity monitors	Summarizing the features of commercially available activity monitors, performance evaluation, and comparison of different activity monitors in terms of different statistical measures	Quantitative in medical applications	Non-vision based	QoS centric	154 (134 key articles out of 2875 articles)

M.J. Kim, 2012 [9]	Identifying significant evaluation methods adapted in user studies of health smart-homes	Listing of system effectiveness evaluation of user studies, analysis of user experience evaluation	Qualitative in medical applications	Vision and non-vision based	QoS centric	41 (20 readable articles in this context out of 82 articles)
T. Tamura, 2012 [11]	Home geriatric physiological and behavioral monitoring approaches	Discussing several sensory devices and appliances, which intend to monitor and assist older adults and disabled people in their living environments	Qualitative in medical applications	Vision and non-vision based	Application centric	91
S. Patel et al., 2012 [12]	Wearable sensors and systems with application in rehabilitation	Summarizing wearable and ambient sensor technology (incl. off-the-shelf solutions) applicable to older adults and subjects with chronic conditions in home and community settings for monitoring health and wellness, safety, home rehabilitation, treatment efficacy, and early detection of disorders	Qualitative in medical applications	Non-vision based	Application centric	124

(continued)

Table 2.1 (continued)

References (first author and year of publication)	Topic	Contents/main contributions	Type of the analysis	Sensors discussed	Viewpoints covered	Number of citations (reviewed works)
M.E. Morris et al., 2013 [3]	Systematic review of smart-home technologies assisting older adults to live well at home	Summarizing studies, which assessed smart-home technologies in terms of effectiveness, feasibility, acceptability, and perceptions of older people	Qualitative in medical applications	Vision and non-vision based	QoS centric	50 (21 out of 1877 key articles included for qualitative synthesis)
P. Rashidi et al., 2013 [4]	Sensors and research projects of ambient assisted living (AAL) tools for older adults	Summarizing emerging tools and technologies for smart-home implementation; classifying the AAL tools and technologies into (a) smart-homes, (b) mobile and wearable sensors, and (c) robotics for supporting ADL, summarizing general sensor types and measurement parameters used in the existing smart-home projects	Qualitative in medical applications	Vision and non-vision based	Technology and application centric	192

A. Cheung et al., 2015 [16]	Systematic literature review of studies, which integrated bedside monitoring equipment to an information system	Gathering evidence on the impact of the patient data management systems (PDMS) on both organizational and clinical outcomes, derived from English articles published between January 2000 and December 2012	Qualitative in medical applications	Non-vision based	QoS centric	39 (18 out of 535 key articles included for qualitative synthesis)
S. C. Mukhopadhyay, 2015 [13]	Reported literature on wearable sensors and devices for monitoring human activities	Summarizing architecture and sensors for human activity monitoring systems, mentioning design challenges for wearable sensors, energy harvesting issues, as well as market trends for wearable devices	Qualitative in both medical and nonmedical applications	Non-vision based	Technology centric	103

of a smart-home technology in the context of monitoring and assisting older adults at home [17], while majority of studies reported on the feasibility of smart-home technology, and other studies were purely observational.

Demiris and Hensel [10] conducted a systematic review of smart-home projects worldwide, discussing applied technologies and models used, categorizing these projects according to different goals, as, for example, the monitoring of physiological vital signs, functional outcomes (e.g., abilities to perform ADLs), safety (e.g., detecting environmental hazards, such as fire or gas leaks) and security (e.g., alerts to human threats), social interactions (i.e., measuring and facilitating human contact including information and communication applications), emergency detection (e.g., falls), and cognitive and sensory assistance (i.e., cognitive aids such as reminders and assistance with deficits in sight, hearing, and touch). They stressed that the design and implementation of informatic applications for older adults should not be determined simply by technological advances but by the actual needs of end users. Furthermore, the current smart-home research needs to address such important questions as health outcomes, clinical algorithms to indicate potential health problems, user perception and acceptance, and ethical implications [10].

In a recent and comprehensive technology- and application-centric surveys, Rashidi et al. [4] summarized the emergence of *ambient assisted living* (*AAL*) tools for older adults based on *ambient intelligence* (*AmI*) paradigm. They summarized the state-of-the-art AAL technologies, tools, and techniques and revealed current and future challenges. They divided the AAL tools and technologies into (a) smart-homes, (b) mobile and wearable sensors, and (c) robotics. They also summarized the general sensor types and measurement parameters used in the smart-home projects.

Another related application-centric article written by Sadri [18] surveyed *AmI* and its applications at home, including care of older adults. The main focus was on ambient data management and artificial intelligence, for example, planning, learning, event-condition-action (ECA) rules, temporal reasoning, and agent-oriented technologies. Sadri found that older adults, typically, need initial training and often follow-up daily assistance, to use *AmI* devices. Finally, security threats as well as social, ethical, and economic issues behind *AmI* were discussed.

One application-centric systematic review by Ali et al. [19] studied specifically gait disorder monitoring using vision and non-vision-based sensors. They showed strong evidence for the development of rehabilitation systems using a marker-less vision-based sensor technology. They therefore believed that the information contained in their review would be able to assist the development of rehabilitation systems for human gait disorders.

Sampaio et al. [20] in his survey on *AmI* made a comparative analysis of some of the research projects, with a specific focus on the human profile, which in the authors' point of view is a crucial aspect to take into account when searching for a correct response to human stimuli. This survey explains both application-centric and QoS-centric matters. The main objective of their work was to understand the current necessities, devices, and the main results in the development of these projects. The authors concluded that most projects do not present the different characteristics and needs of people and miss exploring the potential of human profiles in the context of ambient adaptation.

Another application- and QoS-centric review was conducted by Bemelmans et al. [21], where the authors searched the domain of socially assistive robotics and studied their effects in elderly care. They found only very few academic publications, where a small set of robot systems were found to be used in elderly care. Although individual positive effects were reported, the scientific value of the evidence was limited due to the fact that most research was done in Japan with a small set of robots (mostly off-the-shelf AIBO, Paro [22] and NeCoRo [23]), with small sample sets, not yet clearly embedded in a care need-driven intervention. The studies were mainly of an exploratory nature, underlining the initial stage of robotics as monitoring and assistive technology applied within healthcare.

The recent QoS-centric systematic review by Cheung et al. [16] studied organizational and clinical impacts of integrating various bedside monitoring equipments to an information system, i.e., a computer-based system capable of collecting, storing, and/or manipulating clinical information important to the healthcare delivery process. The authors drew a special attention that implementation of so-called patient data management systems (PDMS) potentially offers more than just a replacement of a paper-based charting and documentation system but also ensures considerable time savings, which can lead to more time left for direct patient care. Additionally, authors concluded that improved legibility, consistency, and structure of information, achieved by using a PDMS, could result in fewer errors.

In one of the most recent technology-centric reviews by Mukhopadhyay [13], the latest reported systems on human activity monitoring based on wearable sensors were discussed, and several issues to tackle related technical challenges were addressed. The author pointed out that development of lightweight physiological sensors could lead to comfortable wearable devices for monitoring different types of activities of home dwellers, while the cost of the devices is expected to decrease in the future.

References

1. Ke, S.R., Thuc, H., Lee, Y.J., Hwang, J.N., Yoo, J.H., Choi, K.H.: A review on video-based human activity recognition. Computers **2**(2), 88–131 (2013)
2. Scanaill, C.N., Carew, S., Barralon, P., Noury, N., Lyons, D., Lyons, G.M.: A review of approaches to mobility telemonitoring of the elderly in their living environment. Ann. Biomed. Eng. **34**(4), 547–563 (2006)
3. Morris, M.E., Adair, B., Miller, K., Ozanne, E., Hansen, R., Pearce, A.J., Santamaria, N., Viegas, L., Maureen, L., Said, C.M.: Smart-home technologies to assist older people to live well at home. J. Aging Sci. **1**(1), 1–9 (2013)
4. Rashidi, P., Mihailidis, A.: A survey on ambient-assisted living tools for older adults. IEEE J. Biomed. Health Inform. **17**(3), 579–590 (2013)
5. Cardinaux, F., Bhowmik, D., Abhayaratne, C., Hawley, M.S.: Video based technology for ambient assisted living: a review of the literature. J. Ambient Intell. Smart Environ. **3**(3), 253–269 (2011)

6. Ludwig, W., Wolf, K.-H., Duwenkamp, C., Gusew, N., Hellrung, N., Marschollek, M., Wagner, M., Haux, R.: Health-enabling technologies for the elderly – an overview of services based on a literature review. Comput. Methods Programs Biomed. **106**(2), 70–78 (2012)
7. Reeder, B., Meyer, E., Lazar, A., Chaudhuri, S., Thompson, H.J., Demiris, G.: Framing the evidence for health smart homes and home-based consumer health technologies as a public health intervention for independent aging: a systematic review. Int. J. Med. Inf. **82**(7), 565–579 (2013)
8. Remoortel, H.V., Giavedoni, S., Raste, Y., Burtin, C., Louvaris, Z., Gimeno-Santos, E., Langer, D., Glendenning, A., Hopkinson, N.S., Vogiatzis, I., Peterson, B.T., Wilson, F., Mann, B., Rabinovich, R., Puhan, M.A., Troosters, T.: Validity of activity monitors in health and chronic disease: a systematic review. Int. J. Behav. Nutr. Phys. Act. **9**(1), 84 (2012)
9. Kim, M.J., Oh, M.W., Cho, M.E., Lee, H., Kim, J.T.: A critical review of user studies on healthy smart homes. Indoor Built Environ. **22**, 260–270 (2012)
10. Demiris, G., Hensel, B.K.: Technologies for an aging society: a systematic review of 'smart home' applications. Yearb. Med. Inform. **47**, 33–40 (2008)
11. Tamura, T.: Home geriatric physiological measurements. Physiol. Meas. **33**(10), R47–R65 (2012)
12. Patel, S., Park, H., Bonato, P., Chan, L., Rodgers, M.: A review of wearable sensors and systems with application in rehabilitation. J. Neuroeng. Rehabil. **9**(1), 21 (2012)
13. Mukhopadhyay, S.C.: Wearable sensors for human activity monitoring: a review. IEEE Sens. J. **15**(3), 1321–1330 (2015)
14. Aggarwal, J.K., Ryoo, M.S.: Human activity analysis: a review. ACM Comput. Surv. **43**(3), 16:1–16:43 (2011)
15. Popoola, O.P., Wang, K.: Video-based abnormal human behavior recognition: a review. IEEE Trans. Syst. Man Cybern. Part C Appl. Rev. **42**(6), 865–878 (2012)
16. Bemelmans, R., Gelderblom, G.J., Jonker, P., Witte, L.: The potential of socially assistive robotics in care for elderly, a systematic review. In: Lamers, M.H., Verbeek, F.J. (eds.) Human-Robot Personal Relationships, vol. 59, pp. 83–89. Springer, Berlin/Heidelberg (2011)
17. Machiko, W.C.M., Tomita, R.: Use of currently available smart home technology by frail elders: process and outcomes. Top. Geriatr. Rehabil. **23**(1), 24–34 (2006)
18. Sadri, F.: Ambient intelligence: a survey. ACM. Comput. Surv. **43**(4), 36:1–36:66 (2011)
19. Ali, A., Sundaraj, K., Ahmad, B., Ahamed, N., Islam, A.: Gait disorder rehabilitation using vision and non-vision based sensors: a systematic review. Bosn. J. Basic Med. Sci. Udruženje Basičnih Med. Znan. Assoc. Basic Med. Sci. **12**(3), 193–202 (2012)
20. Sampaio, D., Reis, L.P., Rodrigues, R.: A survey on ambient intelligence projects. In: 2012 7th Iberian Conference on Information Systems and Technologies (CISTI), pp. 1–6. Madrid (2012)
21. Cheung, A., van Velden, F.H.P., Lagerburg, V., Minderman, N.: The organizational and clinical impact of integrating bedside equipment to an information system: a systematic literature review of patient data management systems (PDMS). Int. J. Med. Inf. **84**(3), 155–165 (2015)
22. Chang, W.-L., Sabanovic, S., Huber, L.: Use of seal-like robot PARO in sensory group therapy for older adults with dementia. In: 2013 8th ACM/IEEE International Conference on Human-Robot Interaction (HRI), pp. 101–102. Tokyo (2013)
23. Nakashima, T., Fukutome, G. Ishii, N.: Healing effects of pet robots at an elderly-care facility. In: 2010 IEEE/ACIS 9th International Conference on Computer and Information Science (ICIS), pp. 407–412. Yamagata (2010)

Chapter 3
Relevant Scenarios for Home Monitoring Solutions for Older Adults

Abstract In this chapter, we describe three common scenarios of older people's living situation in order to increase the understanding of when and how home monitoring can be used among older people at risk of worsening health. We aim at describing the different circumstances under which monitoring approaches and personal care solutions can be applied. Then, we describe relevant geriatric conditions and threats of deteriorating health and functional losses, which are considered to be of paramount need for suitable monitoring solutions. Finally, we summarize these needs in a concise list of conditions and activities that shall be automatically monitored.

Keywords Geriatric conditions • Falls • Delirium • Cognitive impairment • Malnutrition • Multimorbidity • Wandering • Health monitoring scenario • Older adult • Sleeping disorder • Breathing problem • Infection

We acknowledge that older people are individuals with very different health, social, and socioeconomic characteristics, which make them as a whole a very heterogeneous group of the population. Yet we will describe three common scenarios, which we believe cover a majority of the situations encountered by older adults in need of special attention to prevent health deterioration. This includes, but it is not limited to, the description of the involved persons[1] that are receiving or potentially will receive in-home health and personal care. The descriptions may include, for example, the older persons' general health condition (i.e., their physical, mental, and cognitive functional abilities), the current living environment and daily activities, the health-care services and technologies that they already have or are potentially available, and the possible ethical and legal issues. These basic conditions have to be considered before proposing any home monitoring solution. It is important to understand the various scenario descriptions in order to identify the key requirements and needs for an optimal monitoring solution in each single case. For example, the use of video cameras is legally restricted in many countries for privacy reasons, which means that it does not make sense to propose video-based solutions if the legal situation does

[1] In this book we have a primary focus on older adults, mainly aged 70 and over (70+), who are being monitored. Other involved persons may include formal caregivers (nurses, social and health-care assistants, and helpers) and informal caregivers (family, neighbors, and friends).

J. Klonovs et al., *Distributed Computing and Monitoring Technologies for Older Patients*, SpringerBriefs in Computer Science,
DOI 10.1007/978-3-319-27024-1_3

not allow their installation. But even when it is legal, cognitively or mentally impaired persons may not be able or willing to cooperate with caregivers and thus would require other solutions.

Finally, emphasis should be put on establishing seamless and consistent information and communication flow between the different actors in healthcare, i.e., formal home care, general practitioner (family doctor), and secondary healthcare, which requires accessibility to electronic health records (EHR), also for mobile units, to retrieve updated information on health, diseases, and actual treatment, as well as for documentation [1]. Appropriate analysis of which in-home monitoring tools may be used when and where requires principally a broad cooperation between involved engineering teams and healthcare professionals.

The most relevant factors that ultimately influence in-home monitoring scenarios are the older person's conditions and abilities, types of living environment, types of activities, existing infrastructure, current care and medication plans, parameters that need to be monitored, intensity of monitoring, and data transmission, among others.

3.1 Healthy, Vulnerable, and Acutely Ill Older Adults

The older we get, the more diverse we become in terms of health and functions. It is therefore a challenge to categorize older adults into a few descriptive groups and scenarios. Most commonly and depending on the general abilities of older adults, three main groups of in-home monitoring scenarios can be observed: (1) scenarios involving relatively "healthy" older adults, (2) scenarios involving "vulnerable" older adults, and (3) scenarios involving "acutely ill" older adults.

Although the meaning of being healthy can be discussed at length, we describe the main actors of our first scenario as older adults who seem relatively "healthy," as they most likely are independently living in their own home and do not show any particular symptoms of health deterioration [2, 3]. These older adults may still have a few comorbid diseases, e.g., cataract and osteoarthritis, but are not yet hampered in their activities of daily living, although they may have had a few incidents in the past such as falls. Thus, they would benefit from early detection of health-threatening situations and potential risks, e.g., poor lightning at night when they have to go to the bathroom, or fast movements before the body has gained stability, for instance, when rising from a chair. Another monitoring example could be the detection of declining mobility, which may happen, for instance, due to inadequate relief of a bodily pain caused by osteoarthritis in the knee. Less physical activity would lead to a negative spiral with not only worsening of the pain but also disuse of muscles, which in turn leads to muscle wasting and loss of muscle mass and strength, i.e., *sarcopenia*, a disabling disease.

The second scenario type is the most commonly described in the home monitoring literature. It involves "vulnerable" older adults diagnosed with one or more chronic medical conditions [4–10], e.g., chronic obstructive pulmonary disease (COPD), diabetes, cardiovascular diseases, stroke, hypertension, depression, etc., and/or with impaired physical, mental, or cognitive functions. Older adults with chronic diseases are at higher risk of worsening health, e.g., chronic atrial fibrillation increases the risk of getting a stroke and cognitive impairment. Within this scenario, the older persons would in many cases benefit from regular (daily/weekly) attention and possibly assistance from a caregiver. In addition, the monitoring equipment should be adaptable to other requirements for this more vulnerable group of persons, compared to the first scenario, e.g., being applied to older adults who would have difficulties in interacting with the technology but perhaps even accept its presence.

The third scenario type involves older adults, either belonging to the first or the second scenarios, who are developing an acute illness, on top of chronic diseases or conditions, and thus at threat of an acute hospitalization, as exemplified in [8, 11, 12]. This scenario has the most complex requirements for monitoring technology and is often called *hospital at home* (HH) scenario [13]. In addition to monitoring technology, there is usually a need of appropriate assistive technology that makes it feasible for older adults with multiple geriatric conditions to avoid acute admission, or, if admitted to the emergency department, to be discharged earlier to their own dwelling with the appropriate technology.

It is important to note that the aforementioned three main types of scenarios are only rough approximations of patient groups. The boundaries between the three groups are often blurred, while the real-life scenarios would require much deeper insight into the individual patient's characteristics, institutional factors, the current social network situation, the comorbidities, and the main healthcare tasks and goals. Therefore, the next subchapter describes possible geriatric conditions, which are relevant and worthy to have an insight to, in order to understand the challenges of applying in-home monitoring of older adults in their dwellings. Such geriatric conditions would also be involved in the ultimate decision on which type of monitoring devices should be used in one of the three scenarios. Apart from getting insight to the various, but common, geriatric conditions, it is also important to understand that with advancing age the risk of suffering from multiple diseases at the same time increases. Two different words are commonly used when describing disease profiles in older patients: comorbidity and multimorbidity. The first is mainly defined by the coexistence of at least one chronic disease or condition with the disease of interest, while multimorbidity is usually defined as the co-occurrence of at least two chronic conditions within one person at a given time [14]. Multimorbidity is very common within the geriatric population and increases with age [15].

3.2 Relevant Geriatric Conditions and Threats of Deteriorating Health and Functional Losses

This subchapter gives a general brief description of common health conditions and diseases of older adults, focusing on the scenarios of types two and three. Also, we will discuss the most relevant adversities for which monitoring solutions are needed.

We will start with discussing some key terms. With advancing age, older persons undergo some aging-related physical, mental, and cognitive changes, which increase in their vulnerability [16]. The type two scenario of vulnerable older adults may also include, but not only, persons at risk of *frailty*. Frailty has been coined as a state of increased vulnerability to poor resolution of homeostasis after a stressor event, which increases the risk of adverse outcomes, including falls, delirium, and disability [17]. Frailty is a complex condition, which is not only defined by diseases but also by socioeconomic status and social network [18], as well as with an increased level of inflammatory markers [19]. Moreover, frailty is associated with disability and mortality [16, 17], and identifying or detecting some of the factors leading to frailty would be an important scope of *gerotechnology*. As frailty is not only complex but also very common in old age, older people with frailty would benefit from being treated by specialist doctors in *geriatric medicine* or *geriatrics*, which however are underrepresented in many countries despite the demographic challenges of the future [20]. Geriatric medicine is "a branch of general medicine concerned with the clinical, preventative, remedial and social aspects of illness in old age. The challenges of frailty, complex comorbidity, different patterns of disease presentation, slower response to treatment and requirements for social support call for special medical skills." [21]. Consequently, a geriatric patient may be defined as an older person with comorbid conditions and co-occurring functional limitations, in other words, a host of conditions. Further, the geriatric patient is challenging for healthcare professionals because they show atypical symptoms of disease, delaying diagnosis [22–24] and treatment, and, consequently, are at higher risk of developing disability, loss of autonomy, and lower quality of life [25].

In order to keep the autonomy of an older person, the health hazards associated to old age must be addressed from various angles, including the framework of *gerotechnology*, by applying appropriate monitoring technology, which is described in more detail in Chap. 4.

In the reminder of this chapter, we outline and describe the potentially dangerous situations and health threats that occur most frequently in older and very often comorbid and frail patients in our scenarios. We start with discussing falls and injuries in older geriatric patients, since these are among the most frequently reported health problems and serious threats to independent living. Then we review a list of potential health threats, which are the most alarming in the older comorbid population, such as delirium, stroke, hypertension, and heart failure, among others. For each situation, we first define the problem. Then, we discuss its importance and refer to the epidemiology of these occurrences. Finally, we discuss if these problems can be detected, mentioning what data might be necessary to acquire.

For clarity, we are not focusing on diagnostic approaches for major chronic conditions, such as dementia, but rather describing potential adverse events and dangerous situations, which are of potential interest for automated detection.

3.2.1 Falls and Injuries

Across the main three scenario types, falls are very common and may lead not only to injuries and adverse outcomes, such as hip fractures or brain concussions, but also to a secondary effect of fear of falling, which in itself increases the risk of falling and reduced physical activity [26]. As a consequence, social interaction is reduced, loneliness becomes frequent, and quality of life is diminished [27]. A negative spiral may begin and may eventually lead to death, if left unrecognized. Therefore, detection of falls is of paramount importance, not only for identifying those who have fractures or intracranial hematomas but also because many fallers are simply unable to get up by themselves and are therefore at risk of lying on a floor for several hours, even days, with the subsequent risk of dehydration, muscle damage and consequent damage of the kidneys, or even death [28, 29]. Falls could also be the outcome of a stroke or a cardiac arrest. To lower the risk of subsequent further health-threatening complications, fast identification and diagnosis is required.

The adoption of a definition of a fall is an important requirement when studying falls as many studies fail to specify an operational definition, leaving space for interpretation to researchers. This usually results in many different interpretations of falls in the literature [29]. For example, older adults including their family members tend to describe a fall as a loss of balance, while healthcare professionals generally refer to an event which results in a person coming to rest inadvertently on the ground or floor or other lower level leading to injuries and health problems [30, 31].

The geometry of the human body in motion requires an individual to remain balanced and upright under a variety of conditions. Balance is adversely affected by intrinsic and extrinsic factors (). Intrinsic factors are, for example, side effects of medication (e.g., orthostatic hypotension), medical conditions (e.g., stroke), aging-related physiological changes (e.g., declining muscle strength), and nutritional factors (e.g., vitamin D deficiency), while extrinsic factors are, for example, poor lighting conditions, loose carpets, slippery surfaces, stairs, etc. [32, 33]. A systematic review and meta-analysis of risk factors for falls in older adults, who live at home, can be found here [34]. Since in real-life scenarios a great majority of fall incidents in older adults who live alone are not reported to healthcare providers [28], automated detection of falls is of high practical research interest [35].

3.2.2 Delirium

Patients of all three scenarios are potentially at risk of developing delirium, but the more frail and impaired an older person is, the higher is the risk [36]. Delirium is described as an acute confusional state [36]. Delirium may develop as a reaction to infection, dehydration, pain, and painkillers and has a within-hours fluctuating course from cognitively intact to a state of confusion and even agitation (hyperactive delirium), although silent (hypoactive) delirium also occurs [36]. Furthermore, neurological disorders, such as dementia, significantly contribute to the risk of having delirium. Being in an unfamiliar and busy place with many disturbances and strange faces, e.g., a hospital emergency ward, does not enhance recovery in frail older adults, nor does surgery [37]. Some diagnostic tools, such as the Confusion Assessment Method (CAM) [38], are often used to recognize delirium and help distinguish delirium from other forms of cognitive impairment. Treatment should be targeted toward the underlying disease, not the symptoms of delirium, and the delirium will gradually disappear as the initial condition is treated, normally within hours to a few days. Apart from severe causes of delirium, e.g., severe infection, in which intravenous medication is imperative, delirium may not always need to be treated in a hospital setting but may be cared for in the patient's own dwelling if the necessary surveillance can be established. Discharging older persons at risk of delirium to their own home with in-home monitoring soon after establishing a diagnosis and starting targeted treatment will reduce the risk of delirium or shorten the time period of delirium [39].

3.2.3 *Wandering and Leaving Home*

In cases of cognitive impairment, both unrecognized and recognized, the risk of accidents and getting lost while being outdoors (mostly referring to scenario types two and three) can be rather high. A frequent symptom of cognitive impairment and dementia is geographical disorientation, and in more advanced stages, demented persons may leave their dwelling to find their childhood home, a typical delusion of parents being still alive. Such condition may lead to fatal situations, e.g., with wandering in cold weather without proper clothing followed by hypothermia and subsequent death. Therefore, it is important for the caregiver to know whether and when the demented person is leaving the dwelling and, more importantly, when and where wandering behavior may have occurred [40, 41]. However, despite of several attempts to define wandering behavior, no commonly accepted definition of wandering exists so far [42], assumingly because the underlying behavior is very complex and it may present differently depending on the person's physical location (e.g., person's own home, hospital, care facility, or a nursing home). One of the latest and most cited definitions of wandering, proposed by Algase et al. [43], is "a syndrome of dementia-related locomotion behaviour having a frequent, repetitive, temporally disordered, and/or spatially disoriented nature that is manifested in lapping, random, and/or pacing patterns, some of which are associated with eloping, eloping attempts, or getting lost unless accompanied." Detecting and analyzing leaving and returning home habits, as well as travel patterns of older people, are therefore of high importance.

3.2.4 *Malnutrition*

Malnutrition and weight loss are mostly relevant for scenarios two and three but also valid for scenario type 1. Cognitive impairment, loneliness, and depression, as well as poor appetite due to undiagnosed or diagnosed disease or gastrointestinal side effects of commonly used medicines, may lower the appetite of older people and lead to malnutrition and its typical symptom: weight loss. Apart from a geriatric assessment of the etiology of weight loss, securing adequate intake of energy and protein is of paramount importance to revert the otherwise resulting development of sarcopenia (defined previously on Sect. 3.1) and subsequent functional loss. Surveillance of adequate food intake, liquids, and medicine, as well as automated monitoring of body weight, would help to identify older persons at risk of adverse outcomes and thus lead to the initiation of preventive actions. Sarcopenic older persons are at high risk of severe disability, falls, fractures, and institutionalization [44]. It has in recent years been acknowledged that sarcopenia may also be present in obese older adults, so-called sarcopenic obesity, caused by excess intake of energy of poor quality, physical inactivity, and hormonal alterations [45]. Such persons have the same adverse outcomes as low-weight sarcopenic persons and may too benefit from surveillance of adequate food intake.

3.2.5 Sleeping Disorders

Another potential problem, again mostly relevant for scenarios 2 and 3 but also valid for type 1, is disturbances in sleep. In fact, the majority of the geriatric patients experience significant alteration of their sleep patterns and thus overall bad quality of sleep. Changes in sleep pattern are considered to be normal changes with advancing age, with a greater percentage of the night spent in the lighter sleep stages [46, 47], but other causes exist too and can be divided into intrinsic conditions of an individual patient and extrinsic factors related to the environment, where the patient is sleeping. Intrinsic conditions may include pain (e.g., from arthritis), nocturia, medication effects, depression, restless legs syndrome, obstructive sleep apnea (long pauses in breathing associated with snoring), and paroxysmal nocturnal dyspnea (sudden pauses in breathing, experienced during exacerbations of congestive heart failure) [48]. Extrinsic factors may include acoustic noise, lightning, vibration or physical movement, fluctuations of environmental temperature, draught at home, dust, and poor air condition, among others. Thus, monitoring sleep and detecting possible causes of sleep disturbances are of high importance for revealing causes of disturbed sleep.

3.2.6 Shortness of Breath

With advancing age certain physical activities, such as walking upstairs, may cause dyspnea in older adults, who in turn would adapt their physical activities to less challenging activity levels, or even inactivity. Aging is associated to aging-related changes in the respiratory organs leading to lower oxygen uptake from the air to the blood, lower lung volume, and less lung compliance, all leading to shortness of breath when extra respiratory capacity is needed. Diseases such as osteoporotic compression or vertebral deformities of the thoracic vertebras may also affect normal lung function by diminishing the thorax volume [49]. Environmental factors such as smoking and previous employment in jobs associated with dust may reinforce these eventually pathologic changes.

A common medical breathing condition is chronic obstructive pulmonary diseases (abbreviated as COPD), which shares many symptoms with pulmonary emphysema, chronic bronchitis, and asthma. Co-occurring diseases such as chronic heart failure, anemia, and cancers may worsen breathing, as well as acute pneumonia. Also snoring with apnea is considered as a breathing problem, which may lead to lower oxygen intake during sleep and subsequent cognitive impairment [50]. Other reasons of breathing problems may include smoking habits, poor air quality in the living environment, and non-pulmonary infections. Due to the vital importance of pulmonary function, many studies aim at detecting, monitoring, and preventing respiratory problems in older adults at their living environments [51–54].

3.2.7 Hygiene and Infections

Poor hygiene and not the least in combination with a weaker immune system associated to aging may increase the risk of contracting infections, often leading to fever (elevated body temperature). Oral hygiene and oral infections, such as dental caries and oral fungal infections, are important to care about, especially for those individuals who use artificial dentures [55], as it may lead to malnutrition and weight loss and may furthermore cause systemic infections.

Urinary tract infections (UTIs), as another example, can be a serious health threat to older people (). UTIs are common in older adults, especially in women (). Many cases are self-limiting in healthy individuals, but in vulnerable and diseased older persons, a UTI, if untreated, may spread to the blood stream causing systemic infection, kidney damage, delirium, and even death. Common symptoms of UTIs include urgency, frequent and painful urination, and incontinence but may be absent in older adults.

An infection of the lungs (pneumonia) [56] may lead to multiple symptoms, such as cough, fever, shortness of breath, and weakness. The pneumonia may stress the heart and lead to acute heart failure and atrial fibrillation, which further worsens the situation and demands immediate medical attention.

3.2.8 Problems Related to Physical Environment

Finding potential threats in older adult's living environment is relevant for all three scenarios. However, not many studies investigating health conditions of older adults at home were able to thoroughly assess the environmental threats of the older persons' dwellings. For example, levels of environmental noise, lighting, vibrations, ambient temperature, humidity, climate and air condition, and other matters, such as availability of household facilities, can all significantly influence the quality of life of an older individual, especially when the individual suffers from comorbid chronic heart and/or lung conditions. Other environmental hazards may include obstacles in pathways, slippery surfaces, tripping hazards, loose rugs, unsafe or unstable furniture, etc., which may contribute to injuries or falls [57, 58]. Indeed, the most frequently cited causes and risk factors of falls are "accidental" and "environment related," accounting for approximately 30–50 % of all older adult falls [59]. However, many falls attributed to accidents stem from the interaction between identifiable environmental hazards and increased individual susceptibility to such hazards from accumulated effects of ageing and diseases [59].

3.2.9 Underlying Medical Conditions and Multimorbidity

The concept of multimorbidity has been explained earlier and refers to co-occurrence of two or more chronic diseases or conditions within the same individual [14, 15, 60]. Multimorbidity, associated with polypharmacy (i.e., using five or more different medications per day), and adverse side effects of medication increase with advancing age, resulting to more than half of older adults suffering from three or more chronic diseases simultaneously [61]. The most frequent comorbid conditions in older people are [62] hypertension, coronary artery disease, diabetes mellitus, history of stroke, chronic obstructive pulmonary disease, and cancer. Early recognition of acute illness and diagnosis, followed by timely and adequate treatment, is not only the key to prevent severe deterioration in health but also the key to reducing the risk of functional impairments and mortality in geriatric patients. The Comprehensive Geriatric Assessment (CGA) is a tool that has proven effective in terms of reducing mortality and institutionalization [63]. The same principle of comprehensive assessment by monitoring medical parameters and features in older persons at risk, e.g., multimorbid geriatric patients, would be valuable for the individual as well as to the society. However, it requires an understanding of the multidisciplinary nature of health and health deterioration in older adults, and therefore, a broad range of medically sensitive parameters, both objective and subjective, that can detect and measure such deterioration, needs to be considered. Novel automated monitoring technology yet needs to be identified or developed, which will create new perspectives on using in-home monitoring.

3.3 Summary of the Needs

A list of conditions and activities that may be monitored is listed below. The list is far from being exhaustive but addresses the most common needs given by the individual's living style, culture, and acceptance of remote surveillance and monitoring in private homes. The future may bring new conditions, e.g., economic challenges, changed family structures and intergenerational support and care, improved health literacy as well as IT literacy of caregivers, and the target population itself, which may identify new ways of monitoring older adults in their dwellings.

The focus is on the following topics:

- Gait and balance monitoring
- Detecting falls
- Detecting problems related to physical environment
- Detecting wandering
- Detecting delirium
- Recognizing abnormal activity, such as, absence of meal preparation or disturbed day-night cycle
- Monitoring physiological vital status parameters, including body weight
- Monitoring food intake
- Detecting adherence to medication

In the next chapter, we will summarize the available monitoring technologies, which directly or indirectly address and attempt to contribute to the aforementioned topics. Most of these monitoring technologies share common ground as organized in Chap. 4.

References

1. Hägglund, M., Scandurra, I., Koch, S.: Scenarios to capture work processes in shared homecare – from analysis to application. Int. J. Med. Inf. **79**(6), e126–e134 (2010)
2. Botia, J.A., Villa, A., Palma, J.: Ambient assisted living system for in-home monitoring of healthy independent elders. Expert Syst. Appl. **39**(9), 8136–8148 (2012)
3. Naranjo-Hernandez, D., Roa, L.M., Reina-Tosina, J., Estudillo-Valderrama, M.A.: SoM: a smart sensor for human activity monitoring and assisted healthy ageing. IEEE Trans. Biomed. Eng. **59**(11), 3177–3184 (2012)
4. Martín-Lesende, I., Orruño, E., Bilbao, A., Vergara, I., Cairo, M.C., Bayón, J.C., Reviriego, E., Romo, M.I., Larrañaga, J., Asua, J., Abad, R., Recalde, E.: Impact of telemonitoring home care patients with heart failure or chronic lung disease from primary care on healthcare resource use (the TELBIL study randomised controlled trial). BMC Health Serv. Res. **13**(1), 118 (2013)
5. Paré, G., Jaana, M., Sicotte, C.: Systematic review of home telemonitoring for chronic diseases: the evidence base. J. Am. Med. Inform. Assoc. **14**(3), 269–277 (2007)
6. Kim, H., Jarochowski, B., Ryu, D.: A proposal for a home-based health monitoring system for the elderly or disabled. In: Miesenberger, K., Klaus, J., Zagler, W., Karshmer, A. (eds.) Computers Helping People with Special Needs, Proceedings (10th International Conference, ICCHP 2006) Linz, vol. 4061, pp. 473–479. Springer, Berlin Heidelberg (2006)
7. Takahashi, P.Y., Hanson, G.J., Pecina, J.L., Stroebel, R.J., Chaudhry, R., Shah, N.D., Naessens, J.M.: A randomized controlled trial of telemonitoring in older adults with multiple chronic conditions: the tele-ERA study. BMC Health Serv. Res. **10**, 255 (2010)
8. Kang, H.G., Mahoney, D.F., Hoenig, H., Hirth, V.A., Bonato, P., Hajjar, I., Lipsitz, L.A.: In situ monitoring of health in older adults: technologies and issues. J. Am. Geriatr. Soc. **58**(8), 1579–1586 (2010)
9. Pitta, F., Troosters, T., Spruit, M.A., Decramer, M., Gosselink, R.: Activity monitoring for assessment of physical activities in daily life in patients with chronic obstructive pulmonary disease. Arch. Phys. Med. Rehabil. **86**(10), 1979–1985 (2005)
10. Raad, M.W., Yang, L.T.: A ubiquitous smart home for elderly. In: 4th IET International Conference on Advances in Medical, Signal and Information Processing, 2008. MEDSIP 2008, pp. 1–4. Santa Margherita Ligure (2008)

11. Segrelles Calvo, G., Gómez-Suárez, C., Soriano, J.B., Zamora, E., Gónzalez-Gamarra, A., González-Béjar, M., Jordán, A., Tadeo, E., Sebastián, A., Fernández, G., Ancochea, J.: A home telehealth program for patients with severe COPD: the PROMETE study. Respir. Med. **108**(3), 453–462 (2014)
12. Ouslander, J.G., Berenson, R.A.: Reducing unnecessary hospitalizations of nursing home residents. N. Engl. J. Med. **365**(13), 1165–1167 (2011)
13. Morley, A., Sinclair, J.E., Vellas, B.J., Pathy, M.S.J.: Pathy's Principles and Practice of Geriatric Medicine, 2 vols., 5th edn.. Wiley-Blackwell, Chichester/Hoboken (2012)
14. van Oostrom, S.H., Picavet, H.S.J., van Gelder, B.M., Lemmens, L.C., Hoeymans, N., van Dijk, C.E., Verheij, R.A., Schellevis, F.G., Baan, C.A.: Multimorbidity and comorbidity in the Dutch population – data from general practices. BMC Public Health **12**(1), 715 (2012)
15. Barnett, K., Mercer, S.W., Norbury, M., Watt, G., Wyke, S., Guthrie, B.: Epidemiology of multimorbidity and implications for health care, research, and medical education: a cross-sectional study. Lancet **380**(9836), 37–43 (2012)
16. Sieber, C.C.: The elderly patient – who is that?. Internist **48**(11), 1190, 1192–1194 (2007)
17. Andrew Clegg, J.Y.: Frailty in elderly people. Lancet. **381**(9868), 752–762 (2013)
18. Fried, L.P., Tangen, C.M., Walston, J., Newman, A.B., Hirsch, C., Gottdiener, J., Seeman, T., Tracy, R., Kop, W.J., Burke, G., McBurnie, M.A.: Frailty in older adults: evidence for a phenotype. J. Gerontol. A Biol. Sci. Med. Sci. **56**(3), M146–M156 (2001)
19. Collerton, J., Martin-Ruiz, C., Davies, K., Hilkens, C.M., Isaacs, J., Kolenda, C., Parker, C., Dunn, M., Catt, M., Jagger, C., von Zglinicki, T., Kirkwood, T.B.L.: Frailty and the role of inflammation, immunosenescence and cellular ageing in the very old: cross-sectional findings from the Newcastle 85+ study. Mech. Ageing Dev. **133**(6), 456–466 (2012)
20. Kolb, G., Andersen-Ranberg, K., Cruz-Jentoft, A., O'Neill, D., Topinkova, E., Michel, J.P.: Geriatric care in Europe – the EUGMS survey part I: Belgium, Czech Republic, Denmark, Germany, Ireland, Spain, Switzerland, United Kingdom. Eur. Geriatr. Med. **2**(5), 290–295 (2011)
21. Geriatric medicine/Royal college of physicians: https://www.rcplondon.ac.uk/geriatric-medicine (2013). Accessed 12 May 2014
22. Aronow, W.S.: Silent MI. Prevalence and prognosis in older patients diagnosed by routine electrocardiograms. Geriatrics **58**(1), 24–26, 36–38, 40 (2003)
23. Johnson, J.C., Jayadevappa, R., Baccash, P.D., Taylor, L.: Nonspecific presentation of pneumonia in hospitalized older people: age effect or dementia? J. Am. Geriatr. Soc. **48**(10), 1316–1320 (2000)
24. Berman, P., Hogan, D.B., Fox, R.A.: The atypical presentation of infection in old age. Age Ageing **16**(4), 201–207 (1987)
25. Verbrugge, L.M., Jette, A.M.: The disablement process. Soc. Sci. Med. **38**(1), 1–14 (1994)
26. Gill, T.M., Murphy, T.E., Gahbauer, E.A., Allore, H.G.: The course of disability before and after a serious fall injury. JAMA Intern. Med. **173**(19), 1780–1786 (2013)
27. Scheffer, A.C., Schuurmans, M.J., van Dijk, N., van der Hooft, T., de Rooij, S.E.: Fear of falling: measurement strategy, prevalence, risk factors and consequences among older persons. Age Ageing **37**(1), 19–24 (2008)
28. Stevens, J.A.: Falls among older adults – risk factors and prevention strategies. J. Safety Res. **36**(4), 409–411 (2005)
29. World Health Organisation: Global Report on Falls Prevention in Older Age. Geneva (2007)
30. WHO: WHO/Falls. World Health Organisation. http://www.who.int/mediacentre/factsheets/fs344/en/ (2012). Accessed 18 Apr 2014
31. Zecevic, A.A., Salmoni, A.W., Speechley, M., Vandervoort, A.A.: Defining a fall and reasons for falling: comparisons among the views of seniors, health care providers, and the research literature. Gerontologist **46**(3), 367–376 (2006)
32. Samaras, N., Chevalley, T., Samaras, D., Gold, G.: Older patients in the emergency department: a review. Ann. Emerg. Med. **56**(3), 261–269 (2010)
33. Masud, T., Morris, R.O.: Epidemiology of falls. Age Ageing **30**(4), 3–7 (2001)

34. Deandrea, S., Lucenteforte, E., Bravi, F., Foschi, R., La Vecchia, C., Negri, E.: Risk factors for falls in community-dwelling older people: a systematic review and meta-analysis. Epidemiology **21**(5), 658–668 (2010)
35. Igual, R., Medrano, C., Plaza, I.: Challenges, issues and trends in fall detection systems. Biomed. Eng. Online **12**, 66 (2013)
36. Inouye, S.K.: Delirium in older persons. N. Engl. J. Med. **354**(11), 1157–1165 (2006)
37. Freibrodt, J., Hüppe, M., Sedemund-Adib B., Sievers, H., Schmidtke C.: Effect of postoperative delirium on quality of life and daily activities 6 month after elective cardiac surgery in the elderly. Thorac. Cardiovasc. Surg. **61**(S 01), 92 (2013)
38. Waszynski, C.M.: How to try this: detecting delirium. Am. J. Nurs. **107**(12), 50–59 (2007); quiz 59–60
39. Isaia, G., Astengo, M.A., Tibaldi, V., Zanocchi, M., Bardelli, B., Obialero, R., Tizzani, A., Bo, M., Moiraghi, C., Molaschi, M., Ricauda, N.A.: Delirium in elderly home-treated patients: a prospective study with 6-month follow-up. Age **31**(2), 109–117 (2009)
40. Cipriani, G., Lucetti, C., Nuti, A., Danti, S.: Wandering and dementia. Psychogeriatrics **14**(2), 135–142 (2014)
41. Vuong, N.K., Chan, S., Lau, C.T.: Automated detection of wandering patterns in people with dementia. Gerontechnology **12**(3), 127–147 (2014)
42. Lin, Q., Zhang, D., Chen, L., Ni, H., Zhou, X.: Managing elders' wandering behavior using sensors-based solutions: a survey. Int. J. Gerontol. **8**(2), 49–55 (2014)
43. Algase, D.L., Moore, D.H., Vandeweerd, C., Gavin-Dreschnack, D.J.: Mapping the maze of terms and definitions in dementia-related wandering. Aging Ment. Health **11**(6), 686–698 (2007)
44. Cruz-Jentoft, A.J., Baeyens, J.P., Bauer, J.M., Boirie, Y., Cederholm, T., Landi, F., Martin, F.C., Michel, J.-P., Rolland, Y., Schneider, S.M., Topinková, E., Vandewoude, M., Zamboni, M.: Sarcopenia: European consensus on definition and diagnosis report of the European Working Group on Sarcopenia in Older People. Age Ageing **39**(4), 412–423 (2010)
45. Stenholm, S., Harris, T.B., Rantanen, T., Visser, M., Kritchevsky, S.B., Ferrucci, L.: Sarcopenic obesity – definition, etiology and consequences. Curr. Opin. Clin. Nutr. Metab. Care **11**(6), 693–700 (2008)
46. Hägg, M., Houston, B., Elmståhl, S., Ekström, H., Wann-Hansson, C.: Sleep quality, use of hypnotics and sleeping habits in different age-groups among older people. Scand. J. Caring Sci. **28**(4), 842–851 (2014)
47. Namazi, K.H., Chafetz, P.: Assisted Living: Current Issues in Facility Management and Resident Care. Greenwood Publishing Group, Santa Barbara (2001)
48. Crowley, K.: Sleep and sleep disorders in older adults. Neuropsychol. Rev. **21**(1), 41–53 (2011)
49. Lowery, E.M., Brubaker, A.L., Kuhlmann, E., Kovacs, E.J.: The aging lung. Clin. Interv. Aging **8**, 1489–1496 (2013)
50. Engleman, H., Douglas, N.: Sleep 4: sleepiness, cognitive function, and quality of life in obstructive sleep apnoea/hypopnoea syndrome. Thorax **59**(7), 618–622 (2004)
51. Karottki, D.G., Spilak, M., Frederiksen, M., Gunnarsen, L., Brauner, E.V., Kolarik, B., Andersen, Z.J., Sigsgaard, T., Barregard, L., Strandberg, B., Sallsten, G., Møller, P., Loft, S.: An indoor air filtration study in homes of elderly: cardiovascular and respiratory effects of exposure to particulate matter. Environ. Health **12**(1), 116 (2013)
52. Masuda, Y., Sekimoto, M., Nambu, M., Higashi, Y., Fujimoto, T., Chihara, K., Tamura, T.: An unconstrained monitoring system for home rehabilitation. IEEE Eng. Med. Biol. Mag. **24**(4), 43–47 (2005)
53. Chee, Y., Han, J., Youn, J., Park, K.: Air mattress sensor system with balancing tube for unconstrained measurement of respiration and heart beat movements. Physiol. Meas. **26**(4), 413 (2005)
54. Hao, J., Jayachandran, M., Kng, P.L., Foo, S.F., Aung, P.W.A., Cai, Z.: FBG-based smart bed system for healthcare applications. Front. Optoelectron. China **3**(1), 78–83 (2010)

55. Lamster, I.B., Crawford, N.D.: The oral disease burden faced by older adults. In: Lamster, I.B., Northridge, M.E. (eds.) Improving Oral Health for the Elderly, pp. 15–40. Springer, New York (2008)
56. Juthani-Mehta, M., De Rekeneire, N., Allore, H., Chen, S., O'Leary, J.R., Bauer, D.C., Harris, T.B., Newman, A.B., Yende, S., Weyant, R.J., Kritchevsky, S., Quagliarello, V.: Modifiable risk factors for pneumonia requiring hospitalization among community-dwelling older adults: the health, aging, and body composition study. J. Am. Geriatr. Soc. **61**(7), 1111–1118 (2013)
57. Gill, T.M., Williams, C.S., Robison, J.T., Tinetti, M.E.: A population-based study of environmental hazards in the homes of older persons. Am. J. Public Health **89**(4), 553–556 (1999)
58. Northridge, M.E., Nevitt, M.C., Kelsey, J.L., Link, B.: Home hazards and falls in the elderly: the role of health and functional status. Am. J. Public Health **85**(4), 509–515 (1995)
59. Rubenstein, L.Z.: Falls in older people: epidemiology, risk factors and strategies for prevention. Age Ageing **35**(2), ii37–ii41 (2006)
60. Mercer, S.W., Smith, S.M., Wyke, S., O'Dowd, T., Watt, G.C.: Multimorbidity in primary care: developing the research agenda. Fam. Pract. **26**(2), 79–80 (2009)
61. American Geriatrics Society Expert Panel on the Care of Older Adults with Multimorbidity: Guiding principles for the care of older adults with multimorbidity: an approach for clinicians: American geriatrics society expert panel on the care of older adults with multimorbidity. J. Am. Geriatr. Soc. **60**(10), E1–E25 (2012)
62. Akca, A.S.D., Emre, U., Unal, A., Aciman, E., Akca, F.: Comorbid diseases and drug usage among geriatric patients presenting with neurological problems at the emergency department. Turk. J. Geriatr.-Turk Geriatri Derg. **15**(2), 151–155 (2012)
63. Ellis, G., Whitehead, M.A., Robinson, D., O'Neill, D., Langhorne, P.: Comprehensive geriatric assessment for older adults admitted to hospital: meta-analysis of randomised controlled trials. BMJ **343**(1), d6553 (2011)

Chapter 4
Monitoring Technology

Abstract This chapter aims at giving an insight into a variety of available monitoring technologies and techniques, which aim to provide solutions to the issues listed in Chap. 3. First, we start with discussing possible data collection approaches, by revealing choices of available sensors and underlying constrains. Second, we provide a summary of sensors used for data acquisition in regard to needed medical applications, revealing what relevant parameters can be derived from those sensor measurements. We then summarize what common data processing and analysis techniques are used for interpreting this data, with a special focus on machine learning approaches. Third, we derive important requirements and underlying challenges for the involved machine learning strategies and discuss possible implications for applying the different monitoring approaches. Finally, we refer to a number of established standards, which are needed to be complied with, when developing and implementing home monitoring systems for older adults.

Keywords Monitoring technology • Sensor • Physiological parameter • Activity monitoring • Patient at home • Machine learning • Wearable • Remote sensing • Standards • Activity of daily living (ADL)

Most of the smart-home projects, which were briefly introduced in Sect. 1.3, significantly contribute to the research and development of automated monitoring technologies related to the topics listed in Sect. 3.3. Many of these projects proposed holistic approaches, which aim at solving multiple problems simultaneously within one smart-home environment. However, these topics are highly abstracted, and thus, many of them are treated differently, depending on different scenario constraints, on what sensors are applied for data acquisition, and on what information is available a priori. For example, recognition of abnormal activity highly depends on the monitored subset of ADLs, and furthermore, the abnormality may be defined differently. For instance, abnormality may mean a certain deviation from the learned baseline of "normal" everyday activities, or it can be strictly predefined based on prior expert knowledge, e.g., a known sequence of activities that is considered to be abnormal and health threatening.

J. Klonovs et al., *Distributed Computing and Monitoring Technologies for Older Patients*, SpringerBriefs in Computer Science,
DOI 10.1007/978-3-319-27024-1_4

The most common monitoring approach for recognizing health problems at home is motion capture (e.g., for classifying and assessing ADL). Recordings are usually examined manually by healthcare professionals, such as nursing staff, physiotherapists, and occupational therapists, which is very time-consuming [1]. In previous studies about automated monitoring, movement is usually captured using inertial sensors [2], computer vision [3–5], electromyography (EMG) [6], radiofrequency (RF) sensors, or infrared (IR) sensors [7]. For detecting different health threats, video monitoring and computer vision have been widely presented and discussed in the literature, but the main two purposes of these systems were surveillance and communication applications. Video (incl. audio) transmission is usually made in real time over an ordinary telephone line [8] or the Internet [9]. The video can be either viewed directly on a tablet or a monitor by a nurse or doctor, or a video processing system is used to automatically interpret the video data and present the relevant (alarming) information to the medical staff [10] only when some abnormality is detected. The main problem with these video-audio solutions is the ethical issues, i.e., the majority of older adult users are concerned about being monitored by video, as discovered by usability studies, e.g., in the EU-funded Seventh Framework Programme (FP7) Project Confidence [11]. Another common problem is insufficient bandwidth or the quality of Internet connectivity and poor mobile network coverage in some geographic areas such as rural areas. Therefore, it may be impossible to establish real-time video link with sufficiently high resolution of, e.g., complicated wounds, which may need to be treated by a visiting nurse, perhaps guided by a surgeon watching the video in his or her hospital office. Nevertheless, as a communication tool to allow older adults communicating with medical staff on their own request, video-audio technology is already commonly applied [10, 12, 13], when connectivity allows it.

4.1 Sensing and Data Acquisition

There are numerous ways of collecting data about the older persons' health condition, which can be accomplished by asking specific questions and registering answers (considered to be a subjective approach) or by using various sensors (an objective approach). In this book we are mainly interested in collecting objective data, which can be acquired automatically, by using sensors and data capturing devices. However, very often both subjective and objective approaches are combined, to provide as full information as possible.

4.1.1 Types of Sensors and Data Capturing Devices

The different types of sensors used in the field of patient monitoring and the purpose of their employment in regard to the topics listed in Chap. 3 are shown in Table 4.1. The most common purpose of employing these sensors has been for fall detection applications. Fall detectors [54, 107], in most cases, measure motions and accelerations of the

Table 4.1 Summary of sensors used for data acquisition in regard to needed medical applications

Sensor type/sensing modality	Data of interest	Purpose of application	References
Video cameras	Pose estimation, location, movement speed, size and shape changes, custom-defined visual features, temporal semantic data, facial skin color, head motion, face alignment positions	Gait and balance monitoring, fall detection, monitoring the activity of daily living, abnormal activity recognition, activity detection in first-person camera view and detection of activity of taking medicine, measurement of physiological parameters and tracking medical conditions, elopement detection	[14–43]
Microphones	Heart sound, speech, coughing sounds, snoring sounds, stethoscope signal, environmental noise, etc.	Physiological vital status parameter monitoring, environmental threat detection	[44–50]
Infrared (IR) sensors (incl. motion detectors and depth cameras)	Indoor location, movement	Fall detection, abnormal activity recognition, wandering detection	[21, 34, 51, 52]
Accelerometers	Body movement	Fall detection, abnormal activity recognition, wandering detection, gait and balance monitoring, food intake monitoring	[53–63]
Gyroscopes	Body movement, orientation	Fall detection, abnormal activity recognition, gait and balance monitoring	[55, 64–67]
GPS trackers	Outdoor (and limited outdoor) location	Wandering detection	[68, 69]
Pulse oximeter/ near-infrared (cuffless)	SpO_2, blood pressure, heart rate	Physiological vital status parameter monitoring	[39, 44, 70]
Blood pressure monitor (cuffed)	Systolic and diastolic blood pressures and heart rate	Physiological vital status parameter monitoring	[44, 70–77]
Impedance pneumography (IP) sensor	Respiration rate	Physiological vital status parameter monitoring	[78]
ECG device	ECG signal; heart rate; including inter-beat (RR) interval; beginning, peak, and end of the QRS complex; the P and T waves; the ST segment, etc.	Physiological vital status parameter monitoring, arrhythmia detection, delirium detection	[44, 63, 77, 79–81]
EMG device	EMG signal and related parameters	Abnormal activity (incl. inactivity) detection	[63, 77, 82]

(continued)

Table 4.1 (continued)

Sensor type/sensing modality	Data of interest	Purpose of application	References
EEG device	EEG signal, blood glucose levels	Physiological vital status parameter monitoring, detection of various health threats, such as hypoglycemia, epilepsy, sleep apnea, dementia, and other uses	[82–91]
Weighting scale	Body weight	Physiological vital status parameter monitoring, food intake monitoring	[44]
Spirometer	Spirometric parameters, such as forced vital capacity (FVC), peak expiratory flow (PEF), and peak inspiratory flow (PIF)	Physiological vital status parameter monitoring	[44, 92, 93]
Blood glucose monitor	Blood glucose levels	Physiological vital status parameter monitoring	[44, 70, 94, 95]
Pressure mat/carpet	"Step on," "sit on," or "lay on" events	Abnormal activity recognition, wandering detection	[96]
Stove sensor	Stove on/off events	Environmental threat detection	[97]
RFID sensor	Different events (such as taking pills), localization	Abnormal activity recognition, tracking medical conditions, environmental threat detection, food intake monitoring	[98–102]
Temperature sensors	Body temperature, environmental temperature	Physiological vital sign monitoring, detecting problems of physical environment	[63, 69, 77, 103–106]

"Purpose of Application" column refers to detecting health threats for older adults living alone at home, which is relevant to the list specified in Sect. 3.3

person using tags worn around the waist or the upper part of the chest (by using inertial sensors: accelerometers, gyroscopes, and/or tilt sensors). In general, if the accelerations exceed a threshold during a time period, an alarm is raised and sent to a community alarm service. By defining an appropriate threshold, it is possible to distinguish between the accelerations during falls and the accelerations produced during the normal ADL. However, threshold-based algorithms tend to produce false alarms, for instance, standing up or sitting down too quickly often results in crossing a threshold and an erroneous classification of a fall [1]. Several machine learning approaches were also proposed for detection and identification of falls [65, 108–111], which help to minimize those false alarms by automatically adapting to specifics of the monitored person. The use of indoor localization sensors (both IR and RF based) has also been reported [109, 112], which are intended for localizing persons in 3D space and analyzing their movements, useful for detecting accidental falls or abnormal activity.

Another common technology for fall and/or accident detection is emergency alarm systems, which usually include a device with an alarm button [98, 113], e.g., embedded in a mobile phone, pendant, chainlet, or a wristband. These devices can be used to alert and communicate with a responsible care center. However, such devices are efficient only if the person consciously recognizes an emergency and is physically and mentally capable to press the alarm button. Also static alarm buttons exist, which are often placed in the toilet or bathroom, as required by the BS 8300 and ISO 21,542 standards [114, 115].

The sensors reported in the literature included (but were not limited to) infrared (IR) and near-infrared (NIRS) sensors [21, 103, 116–120], video [15, 42, 121] and thermal cameras [122, 123], bioelectrical sensors (used in ECG, EMG, EEG) [63, 80, 81, 124, 125], ultrasonic sensors and microphones [126–130], radiofrequency (RF) transceivers, piezoresistive and piezoelectric sensors [131–133], inertial sensors (such as accelerometers, gyroscopes, and tilt sensors) [53, 54, 56–60, 63–65, 134], electrochemical sensors (such as smoke detectors, CO_2 meters, blood glucose and hemoglobin testers) [135–139], as well as mechanical measurement devices (such as weighing scales).

Video cameras and thermal cameras have two different types: static cameras and active PTZ (pan-tilt-zoom) cameras. IR sensors also have two types, active and passive, but the meaning of activeness in this context is different. Instead of being able to rotate or zoom in and out, active IR sensors emit IR radiation pattern and then capture the reflection of the infrared rays. On the other hand, passive IR (i.e., PIR) sensors merely capture the IR radiation from the environment. Ultrasonic sensors, for instance, are typically active, meaning that an ultrasound transmitter is involved and an ultrasound receiver is tuned to capture the reflected ultrasonic waves initially emitted by the transmitter.

Bioelectrical sensors measure electrical current generated by a living tissue. Electrochemical sensors typically measure the concentration of the substance of interest (such as gas or liquid), by chemically reacting with that substance and consequently producing an electrical signal proportional to the substance concentration. Piezoresistive sensors measure changes in the electrical resistivity of a piezoresistive material (e.g., consisting of semiconductor crystals) when a mechanical stress is applied to it. On the other hand, piezoelectric sensors measure the electrical potential generated by a piezoelectric material itself, which is also caused by applying mechanical force to it.

Most of these aforementioned sensors have been utilized for data acquisition in different areas of older patient monitoring, such as activity of daily living (ADL), instrumental activity of daily living (IADL), abnormal activity detection such as fall detection or wandering, and extraction of physiological parameters.

Hence, the general goal of using the aforementioned sensors is to measure relevant physical properties for estimating specific medically important parameters (often called as *biosignals* or *biomarkers*), which are summarized in Sect. 4.1.3 and which allow to further infer the patients' health conditions [140] followed by manual or automatic analysis (Fig. 4.1).

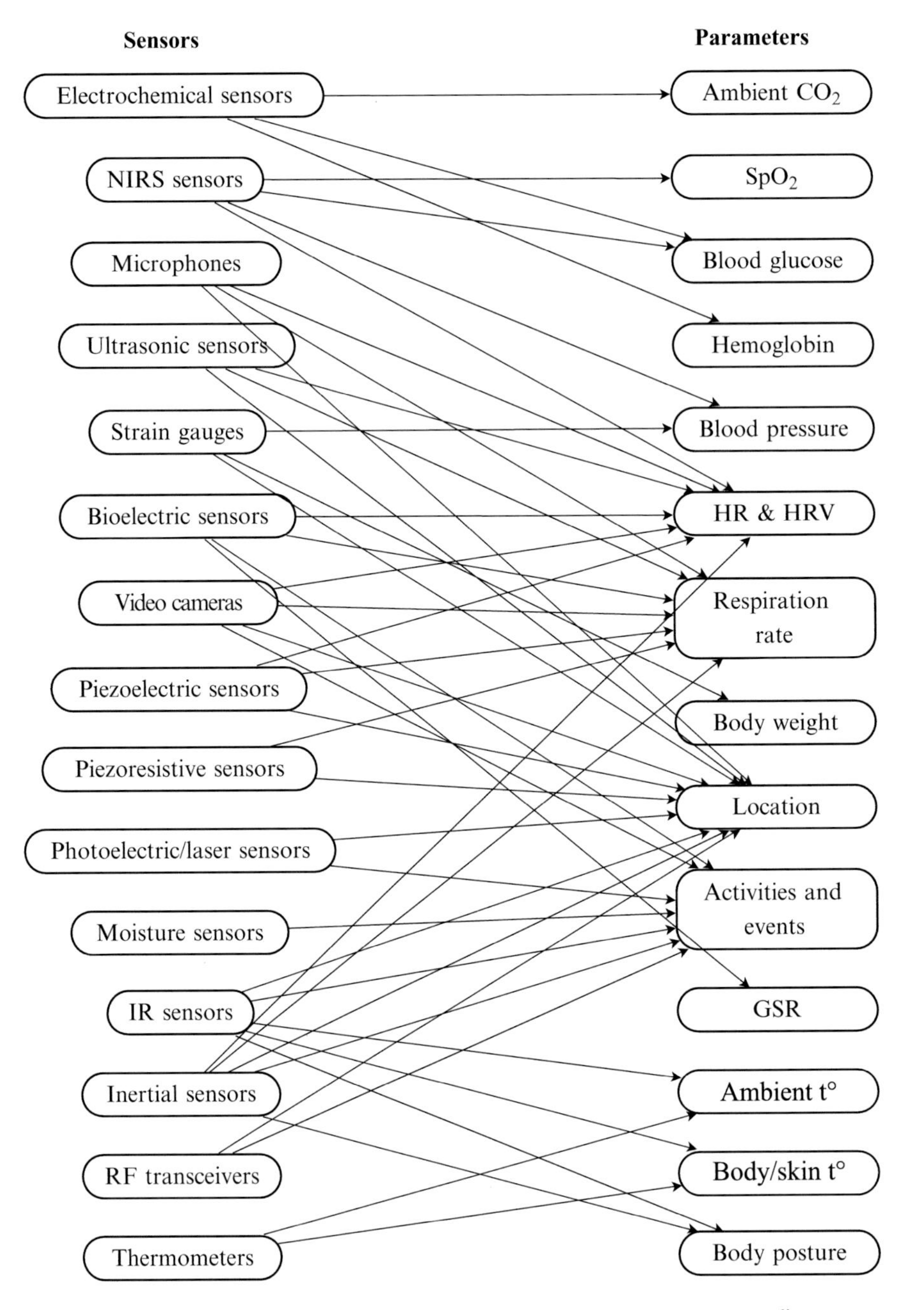

Fig. 4.1 The linkage between the identified sensors and the most common corresponding parameters (summarized in Sect. 4.1.3), which can infer patients' health conditions and therefore can be valuable assets for each of the three scenarios (introduced in Chap. 3). *NIRS* stands for near-infrared spectroscopy, *IR* infrared, *RF* radiofrequency, CO_2 carbon dioxide (concentration), SpO_2 peripheral capillary oxygen saturation, i.e., estimation of the oxygen saturation level, *HR* and *HRV* stand for heart rate and heart rate variability, respectively, *GSR* galvanic skin response, *t°* temperature

4.1.2 Sensor Location and Placement

Technically, there are infinite location options for placing the variety of sensors intended for in-home monitoring. The choice of these sensors and their placement, however, highly depends on the needs seen by patients and medical staff, on physical and mental conditions of a person, who needs to be monitored, and on the various scenario constrains, including existing infrastructure options, physical layout of the dwelling, etc. In general, these sensors can be divided in the following groups in terms of their placement:

1. *On-body sensors*, such as skin patches and sensors worn by an individual as an accessory or embedded in the outfit (part of clothing), like:

   (a) Electronic skin patches or artificial skin, as exemplified in [52, 141, 142], that can be glued to the skin on a body area of interest and which may include various sensors for measuring various physiological parameters, such as (but not limited to) body temperature, heart rate, EMG parameters, pulse oximetry for monitoring the oxygen saturation (SpO_2), as well as accelerometers, moisture sensors, and possibly others.
   (b) Wristwatches, wristbands, and armbands [103, 143–147] or rings [103, 148], measuring heart rate, body temperature, near-body ambient temperature, galvanic skin response (GSR), and EMG data. Similarly, these sensors can also be incorporated into jewelry, such as necklaces, brooches, pins, earrings, belt buckles, etc.
   (c) Clothes, belts, and shoes for monitoring gait, motion, and vital signs and detection of health emergencies [133, 149]. The most common are chest-worn belts and "smart textile" shirts for measuring vital signs and motion [78, 131, 133, 150, 151]. Other examples may include gloves for recording finger and wrist flexion during ADLs and/or vital signs [152, 153], a waist-band with textile sensors for measuring acidity (pH levels) of sweat and sweat rate [139], or moisture-sensitive diapers [154].
   (d) Headbands and headsets for monitoring brain activity, based on EEG and NIRS signal analysis [82, 155, 156].

2. *Remote sensors*, which can be placed on ceilings or desks, embedded in pieces of objects, furniture, in the floor of a house, which are usually static (i.e., not mobile). These can include the following:

   (a) Sensors, which are mounted on ceilings or walls (incl. corners), include video cameras (with or without microphones); [21, 42, 121, 125] IR active and passive sensors (including thermal imaging) [118–120, 122, 144, 157, 158], and ultrasound sensor arrays [159]. Those sensors are used mainly for localization and motion capture of home residents and also for measuring various physiological signs, such as breathing rate and cardiac pulse, as well as for assessing functional status of older adults at home; detecting emergencies, such as falls; and recognizing various ADLs. Noteworthy, the majority of the aforementioned monitoring approaches do not require wearing tags or carrying a mobile device for older persons during monitoring; however, several IR-based motion capture systems [66, 160] and RF-based localization systems [11, 109, 161, 162] do require wearing dedicated tags or *on-body* devices attached to a subject and thus are mainly meant for experimental purposes.

(b) Pressure-sensitive mats, carpets, beds, sofas, and chairs, or load-sensing floor, which are used for monitoring movement, assessing gait, detecting falls, and recognizing sitting and sleeping postures, as well as ADLs [163–168]. Various contextual data can be extracted from load-sensing techniques, for example, the body weight or position of a person. Other sensors, such as moisture sensors, can be also embedded into bed mattresses or sofas, to detect, for example, possible urinary incontinence [132, 169], or vibration sensors, embedded in the floor, for movement tracking and fall detection [170].

(c) Ambient temperature, humidity, CO_2 concentration, vibration, particle, lightning sensors, microphones, and smoke detectors, which are placed in all or certain rooms of older residents, to monitor environmental living conditions, to recognize different ADLs, as well as to screen for certain emergencies [48, 94, 105, 171–173]. Usually these sensors are also mounted on walls or ceilings.

(d) Medication tracking and reminder systems, as well as usage tracking of different items at home, usually based on RFID technology [31, 101, 102]. These systems could detect how many times an older adult uses his or her preferred items, thus providing a good measure of the person's ADLs.

3. *Implantable* (in vivo) *devices*, like:

   (a) Implantable cardiac monitors, i.e., ECG loop recorders [174]
   (b) Smart pills, e.g., for gastric pressure and pH level measurement [175]
   (c) Continuous glucose-monitoring biosensors, e.g., implanted into the inner ear of subjects, detecting hypoglycemia from EEG signals [84, 90]
   (d) Wireless capsule for endoscopy [176]

4. *Portable (mobile) devices*, like:

   (a) Smartphones and tablets [38, 57, 60, 64, 134, 152, 177–179]
   (b) Multimedia devices or systems [94, 180, 181]
   (c) Robots equipped with multimodal sensors [125, 180, 182–185]
   (d) Portable video cameras and microphones [10, 186]

For a number of practical and financial reasons, the devices mentioned in the fourth group of the above list are often used as devices for the first and second group. Furthermore, smartphones and tablets typically provide wider range of functionality, including transmission, storage, processing, accessing of the data and relevant information, as well as providing functionality for human-computer interaction.

Systematic evaluation is needed in order to quantify which location and placement is the most suitable for the sensors. For instance, Kaushit et al. [63] evaluated the characteristics of a pyroelectric infrared (PIR) detector to identify any section of a room, where the detector will fail to respond, and assessed the number of detectors required to identify reliably the movements of the occupant. They showed the spatial characteristics of PIR detector and assessed the minimum number of detectors required to sense even small movements (e.g., reading a book) in its defined field of view in order to monitor activities of older people living alone at home. They suggested combining several detectors (four per room – one at each corner of the room) in order to gather reliable data for all types of movements to assess the occupancy patterns of the room, because a single detector was not capable of providing information about the level of activity performed by the occupant.

One of the most promising patient monitoring technologies is based on health monitors that are body worn (e.g., on the wrist). Most commonly, they are intended to continuously monitor the pulse, skin temperature, movement [187–191], and other data of interest. Usually, at the beginning of the systems usage, the pattern for the user is learned. For this purpose, machine learning approaches are used (see Sect. 4.2.1). Afterwards, if any deviations are detected, alarms are typically sent to the emergency center. Such a system can detect various health threats, for example, collapses, faints, blackouts, etc. The drawbacks of these systems are poor tracking accuracy [11] and that people are not likely to carry the body-worn devices at all times, even if the transceiver is built into a convenient form, such as a wristwatch, a smartphone, or a bracelet.

Finally, the common problem with most of the currently proposed health monitoring systems is that patients are often compelled to wear or even carry on uncomfortable and/or cumbersome equipment, to be within certain smart-home rooms or beds fitted with monitoring devices, which clearly restricts older persons' activity [192]. The challenge of building monitoring system, which can automatically monitor older patients at home and detect dangerous conditions and situations, remains unsolved. In order to solve the abovementioned problems, it is strategically important to prioritize the most unobtrusive technological solutions with a trade-off of capturing enough *clinically useful* data.

4.1.3 Summary of Parameters

All sensible parameters can be categorized into the five main classes, which represent the nature of the target measures:

1. Physiological parameters, as, for example, in [193–199], which represent intrinsic functioning of human body (often called as vital signs) such as pulse, blood pressure, respiration rate, temperature, lung vital capacity, blood oxygenation, blood glucose levels, hemoglobin, cholesterol, blood lactate, and others

2. Behavioral parameters, as, for example, in [3, 64, 107, 192, 196, 197, 200–203], which can be observed extrinsically (e.g., represented as ADL, cognitive tasks, social interaction, etc.)
3. Parameters describing sensory, cognitive, and functional abilities of a person [204–206], e.g., strength and balance, that can be measured, for instance, through a "handgrip" test and a balance tests, respectively, or other physical and cognitive parameters, which can be assessed by performing specific ADLs
4. Anthropometric parameters [53, 207] (such as weight and height, body circumferences, body mass index, and knee-heel length), which usually stay constant and are necessary for statistical comparison between diversity of older adults, and in some cases, detecting a body weight loss or gain may be of interest
5. Environmental parameters [94, 169, 208–212] (such as ambient temperature, humidity, pressure, lighting, environmental noise, air quality, etc., which are important factors for health condition)

In general, human health state can be defined by a variety of physiological and behavioral parameters, which usually are self-interdependent. However, not all of them are equally important, and not all of those parameters can be easily and precisely measured, requiring different medical equipment and measuring approaches (e.g., invasive, noninvasive, and distance monitoring).

From the reviewed works, it is evident that only few studies covered two or more aspects simultaneously, and no work was found where all the five sensor categories were considered. In practice, there are obvious overlaps between what sensory technology is used, what biosignals are measured, and how and where they are measured. By applying sensor fusion techniques, it is possible to:

1. Make the sensors work in equilibrium (i.e., synchronized in time and cross dependent, when one or more measured parameters can rectify another parameter of interest being monitored, as described by the heterogeneous approach [213])
2. Optimally select the hardware, with the aim of achieving maximally accurate, complete, and consistent patient records

In the related works, optimality of sensor selection is generally assessed by the following measures that might play a role in different scenarios:

1. Validity and reliability of the sensor measurements. Validity refers to the degree to which a measurement method or instrument actually measures the concept in question and not some other concept. It often refers to precision and accuracy of a monitored parameter measured by a sensor or estimated by a sensor system. Reliability refers to the degree to which a sensor or a sensor system produces stable and consistent data over time. For example, it should be stable to noise and robust to patient's activity and location [189].
2. Comfortability, which is often measured based on the nonintrusiveness and noninvasiveness of sensors [214, 215]. For example, on-body noninvasive sensors are more feasible for home appliances than invasive ones, while a remote unobtrusive (distance monitoring) approach is more comfortable than, e.g., wearable/

on-body sensors. Size, form, and weight are also considered as important factors for the comfortability measure of wearable sensors [113]. Hensel et al. [214] describe in total eight different types of user-perceived obtrusiveness that are caused by home telehealth technology and which should be considered when evaluating comfortability.
3. Durability and longevity, which describes how long a particular device can operate, in terms of wear and tear and in case of necessity to change some parts, such as stickers or patches [216].
4. Energy efficiency, which is assessed in terms of energy consumption and battery life [216, 217].
5. Observation ranges and location and placement of sensors, which ultimately defines whether or not it is feasible to use the sensors under certain constraints and how many sensory devices should be used [218]. In addition, the effects of potential sensor displacement should be considered as well [219].
6. Low cost, which justifies the financial feasibility for applying the proposed sensors [166].

4.2 Data Processing and Analysis

In this subchapter we review the available methods for analyzing, using, and understanding the data collected by the sensors described in the previous chapter.

4.2.1 Machine Learning Approaches

Machine learning techniques are able to examine and to extract knowledge from the monitored data in an automatic way, which facilitates robust and more objective decision-making. Although the number of potential applications for machine learning techniques in geriatric medicine is large, few geriatric doctors are familiar with their methodology, advantages, and pitfalls. Thus, a general overview of common machine learning techniques, with a more detailed discussion of some of these algorithms, which were used in related works, is presented in this chapter.

Numerous recent studies [64, 91, 198, 220–230] have attempted to leverage different machine learning techniques on a wide variety of data readings to solve problems of detecting potential health threats automatically and to better understand health conditions of older adults at their living environment. Most of the discussed problems are concerned with classification tasks, as, for example, where the desired result is a categorical variable, i.e., a class label [15, 17, 19, 65, 66, 220, 228–238]. The most notable examples of classification tasks are fall detection [15, 17, 19, 65, 228, 232, 234, 237, 238] and abnormal behavior or event detection [220, 229, 233] (which can be caused, for instance, by falls or health deterioration) in older adults. Few other works are solving regression problems, like in [239–241], where the goal is to estimate a continuous variable. Regression examples include predicting functional ability [239], estimating mortality risk in geriatric patients [240], or continuously estimating a vital sign, such as blood pressure or blood glucose concentration [70], based on other noninvasively measurable parameters. It is important to note that regression is often used as an intermediate step before final classification, as, for example, in [234, 242–245], where a continuous regression curve is truncated into two distinct classes or more (most commonly ordinal) categories. It is worthy to mention that sometimes a regression curve is also used to estimate a boundary that explicitly separates two classes, but there are no relevant studies yet, where it is mentioned in our context. For instance, logistic regression can be often used as a classifier.

There are numerous works, which report treating the posed problems in a *supervised* fashion, when a dataset with empirical data including correct classification or regression results is provided as a "learning material" for training and testing machine learning techniques, as, for example, in studies dealing with recognizing ADLs [22, 25, 26, 30, 246–248], where datasets with clear labels for each activity annotated by a human expert were used. Most of these studies focus purely on the detection of "alarming situations" (e.g., a fall) commonly treated in *discriminative* fashion, i.e., learning to distinguish an alarming event from non-harmful situations based purely on the previously monitored data and finding dependency of annotations (ground truth). These problems can be solved by *discriminative* (often called as *conditional*) models, such as by logistic regression [234, 243, 245], support vector machines (SVMs) [59, 228, 242, 249, 250], conditional random fields [30, 230, 247, 251, 252], boosting [253], and artificial neural networks (ANNs) [254, 255]. Often researchers simplify the problem as a *binary* classification, by considering only two classes, for instance, classifying "an alarming situation" versus "a non-alarming situation" (usually applied in short-term monitoring scenarios, e.g., fall detection) or diagnosing a certain impairment (usually applied in long-term monitoring scenarios, e.g., dementia diagnosis). However, many recent studies attempted solving *multi-class* classification problems, i.e., distinguishing between more than two classes, for instance, in the scenarios, where multiple ADLs are recognized [21, 22, 30, 247, 256, 257]. Binary classification approaches are relatively easy to evaluate, compared to multi-class classification methods.

Furthermore, hierarchical classification models exist, which are useful for distinguishing activities or events on different abstraction levels. For example, at first, a fall or a non-fall is classified; then in case of a non-fall, a more specific activity is then returned; and in case of a fall, the type of fall is further estimated [22, 65, 120]. These hierarchies can be learned and represented as decision trees (DTs) [22] or random forests [47]. By default, some of the discriminative approaches, such as logistic regression, SVMs, or ANNs, can output only a discrete class label for a given sample, while some can provide a probabilistic estimate of a sample being a part of either class, such as CRFs. Thus, in patient-at-home scenarios, when geriatric care requires a probabilistic measure representing a likelihood of a detected health threat, probabilistic approaches are more preferable [258]. This can be accomplished also by applying several *generative models* (often referred to *probabilistic classification*), such as naïve Bayesian classifier (NBC) [220], dynamic Bayesian networks (DBN) [16, 259, 260], hidden Markov models (HMMs) [58, 201, 230, 261], Gaussian processes (GPs) [262–264], Gaussian mixture models (GMMs) [16, 263, 265], or deep belief networks [266]. GPs proved to be very effective in the patient monitoring scenarios both for solving regression [260, 267] and for classification [16, 259] tasks. Like SVMs, GPs are kernel methods. GPs, proved to handle well multidimensional inputs and unequally sampled data points, have a relatively small number of tuneable parameters that does not require lots of training data. However, choosing the right kernel function is a question of experience. Difference between other discriminative and generative models in the light of activity recognition has been discussed in [30].

Popular graphical models, such as Markov chains, dynamic Bayesian networks [16, 30, 241, 259, 260, 268, 269], hidden Markov models (HMMs) [58, 201, 230, 261], and conditional random fields (CRFs) [30, 230, 247, 252, 269, 270], are reported to deal successfully with the sequential nature of data. HMMs are the most common graphical models for activity recognition, and many extensions have been proposed, for example, the coupled HMM for recognizing multi-resident activities, hierarchal HMM for providing hierarchal definitions of activities, hidden semi-Markov model for modeling activity duration, and partially observable Markov decision process for modeling sequential decision processes.

There are also several works, which treat problems in an *unsupervised* fashion (without knowing “correct” answers a priori), when the task is to automatically discover structure or new patterns in given data, and therefore, clustering and/or outlier analysis is used [33, 35, 55, 223, 229, 253]. Unsupervised and supervised learning is often used in conjunction, when clustering results serve as an extra input for classification, as, for example, in [55, 253]. For instance, in [55] clustering was used for revealing an uncommon acceleration that potentially indicated a fall, which was used as an input for a classifier; while [253] demonstrated the use of unsupervised classification for amplifying predictability of models describing expert classification of coronary heart disease (CHD) patients, as well as boosting cause-and-effect relationships hidden in the data. As an example of a relatively simple technique, k-means algorithm itself is often used to initialize the parameters in a Gaussian mixture model before applying the *expectation maximization* algorithm [271], p. 427. There are also other ways, where a number of studies reported the application of *unsupervised* machine learning approaches for improving the performance of health-threatening event detection systems. For example, Yuwono et al. [55] used the data stream from a waist-worn wireless triaxial accelerometer and combined the application of discrete wavelet transform, regrouping particle swarm optimization, Gaussian distribution of clustered knowledge, and an ensemble of classifiers, including a multilayer perceptron and augmented radial basis function (ARBF) neural networks. Clustering was used for revealing an uncommon acceleration that potentially indicated a fall, which was used as an input for a classifier.

4.2.2 Requirements and Challenges of Machine Learning Strategies

The types and distributions of monitored data dictate the specific requirements for machine learning techniques that intend to handle and reason from these data. For example, the following requirements for machine learning techniques that intend solving medical-related tasks can be noted [272]:

1. Good performance (e.g., high accuracy and precision)
2. Dealing with missing data (e.g., loss of some amount of data should not result in a rapid drop of performance)
3. Dealing with noisy data (e.g., when some errors in data are present)
4. Dealing with imbalanced data (e.g., when class distribution is not uniform among the classes of interest)
5. Dealing with uncertainty (e.g., when imprecision, vagueness, or gradedness of training data is present)
6. Transparency of diagnostic knowledge (i.e., the automatically generated knowledge and the explanation of decisions should be transparent to the responsible medical personnel, possibly providing a novel point of view on the given problem, by revealing interrelation and regularities of the available data in an explicit form)
7. Ability to explain decisions (e.g., the process of decision-making of a machine learning approach should be transparent to the user. For instance, when a certain health threat is automatically detected, an algorithm should present an explanation of the circumstances, which forced to make such a statement. For example, graphical models and decision trees are more acceptable than so-called black box algorithms, where mathematical reasoning is hardly explainable to the responsible medical personnel.)
8. Ability to reduce a number of tests without compromising the performance (since the collection of patient data is often expensive and time-consuming for the patients, it is desirable to have a classifier that is able to reliably detect a certain health threat with a relatively small amount of training data about the target patients. A machine learning approach should be able to select an appropriate subset of attributes during the learning process.)
9. Dealing with growing dimensionality (e.g., adding new sensors may provide additional information about a given problem; thus, a machine learning approach should be able to accept extra measurements or new parameters as an input; and the decision-making should be susceptible to this input after classifier retraining.)
10. Continuously learn (and improve) from new data (i.e., when new empirical data is available, a machine learning approach should be able to relearn from the new input. For example, so-called *active learning* approaches may be applied [273].)

In most cases, the performance of a classifier (e.g., a fall detector) is expressed in terms of sensitivity and specificity. For example, in the case of a binary classifier, the sensitivity is the ability of a detector to correctly classify a fall event as a fall, while the specificity is the ability of a detector to correctly classify normal activity as being normal. In other words, sensitivity represents the percentage of how well the algorithm detects a certain event or activity when that event or activity actually occurred (i.e., positive cases), while specificity represents the percentage of how well the algorithm can rule out all other events or activities than the one that is being identified (i.e., negative cases). Another commonly used performance measure is classification accuracy, which represents the percentage of the correctly classified events or activities among all events or activities that are being observed (both positive and negative cases). It is important to note that accuracy measure alone is not enough for assessing the overall performance of the classifier, because it does not reveal how well the classifier can detect an important health threat of interest. For example, if a dataset contains very few instances of positive cases, comparing to the number of negative cases, and the algorithm is tuned to classify all instances as negative cases (i.e., the sensitivity is 0), then the accuracy can still be very high (close to 100 %), which would be obviously misleading, because such algorithm would not be capable of detecting the important health threat at all.

Throughout a variety of technical articles on solving medical issues, one can easily stumble upon ill-posed problems. For example, the potential problem of class overlap (when a sample is a part of either class simultaneously) is often neglected in the technical articles, which can lead to false evidence with unsubstantiated results. For instance, in [66] the authors attempted to classify a user's gait into one of the following five classes: (1) normal, (2) with hemiplegia, (3) with Parkinson's disease, (4) with pain in the back, and (5) with pain in the leg. However, in a real-world scenario, these classes can potentially overlap (for instance, people may experience pain in the back and in the leg at the same time); therefore, the classification results should not be generalized, and the trained (discriminative) classifier models might not be appropriate, especially when healthy young individuals were used to simulate the gait for each class. This, however, is a general design problem of testing protocols.

More complex examples of classification problems include both the situations with naturally overlapping classes and, furthermore, the situations when the uncertainty of the ground truth is high. These problems are sometimes called as continuous classification problems, and the data behind such problems is often referred to fuzzy sets. When it is combined with problems, such as class imbalance (when the total number of available data instances of one class is far less than the total number of data instances of another class), which is implicit in most of the real-world applications, the situation becomes even more complicated. Recent works [274, 275] prove that the successful trick to deal with class imbalance problems is to include additional pre-processing steps, such as undersampling and oversampling methods, e.g., "synthetic minority oversampling technique" (SMOTE) [276], which oversamples the minority class by creating "synthetic" samples based on spatial location of the samples in the Euclidean space. A recent approach by Das et al. [275] was able to more accurately distinguish individuals with mild cognitive impairment (minority class) from healthy older adults (majority class), by applying so-called ClusBUS (a clustering-based undersampling technique). This technique successfully identified data regions, where minority class samples were embedded deep inside majority class. By removing majority class samples from these regions, ClusBUS preprocessed the data in order to give more importance to the minority class during classification, which outperformed existing methods, such as SVM, C4.5 DT, kNN, and NBC, for handling class overlapping and imbalance.

Among the proposed approaches, there was a high ambiguity in the definitions of the classes, as well as different training and test datasets were used, and the reported machine learning algorithms have highly varying complexities [55, 66, 109, 234, 252, 269, 277]. Therefore, comparing the performances of these diverse algorithms is fundamentally not feasible in an objective manner, unless benchmarking datasets and well-defined evaluation strategies are used. For example, Khawandi et al. [237] proposed an algorithm of learning using a decision tree for fall detection based on the simultaneous input from a video camera and a heart rate monitor, which showed a low error rate of 1.55 % in average on test data after training. However, no definition of a falling event was revealed, and a description of the used dataset and the learning speed of the algorithm were missing.

It is important to note that every machine learning strategy has some limitations. For example, Zhang et al. [59] proposed a fall detector based on support vector machine (SVM) algorithm, which used input from one waist-worn accelerometer. The features for machine learning were the accelerations in each direction and changes in acceleration, and their method detected falls with a promising 96.7 % accuracy. Despite that SVMs are relatively fast and efficient to compute, they do not output with what probability a sample belongs to either class. Other well-known limitations of SVMs are a choice of the kernel function and high algorithmic complexity.

In order to avoid some limitations of individual machine learning approaches and consequently to improve the overall classification or regression performances, multiple learning methods can be used at the same time, called as ensemble methods. They use multiple learning algorithms to obtain better predictive performance than could be obtained from any of the constituent learning algorithms. Therefore, ensemble methods are increasingly attractive for research on problems of monitoring older patients [43, 226, 240, 278]. Furthermore, it is often favorable to use a set of relatively simple learners, which can result in a better performance, comparing to a single complex and computationally expensive method.

For combining the above machine learning techniques in an effective manner, one should be extremely careful, because there are a number of different learning stages, and different learning problems are addressed, so that incorrect treatment of data can accumulate and result in false reasoning. As previous research suggests, for optimal results, a physician or clinical expert will only be able to guide and understand the research if it possesses sufficient basic knowledge of the machine learning algorithms [279].

Meanwhile, some recent studies have further attempted to compare the performances of machine learning systems with human experts. For example, Marschollek et al. [243] compared the performances of a multidisciplinary geriatric care team with automatically induced logistic regression models based on conventional clinical and assessment data as well as matched sensor data. Their results indicated that a fall risk model based on accelerometer sensor data performs almost as well as a model that is derived from conventional geriatric assessment data.

4.3 Standards

Generally, a wide variety of monitoring technologies for older patients, i.e., the sensory devices, including software, are considered to fall under the definition of a "medical device." A full definition of a "medical device" by World Health Organization is given here [280]. Medical devices are considered to be a subset of electronic products that may have general regulatory provisions [281]. Numerous national and international standards exist that must be complied with before and after such electronic products enter into commercial use. These standards offer a possibility to cope with the high demands on technical and scientific expertise in the regulation processes of medical devices. These standards are being constantly updated, following the high rate of innovations.

It is important to note that medical devices may be regulated even for nonmedical reasons. For example, if the device (an electronic product) emits or can potentially emit some type of electronic product radiations, such as x-rays and other ionizing radiation; ultraviolet, visible, infrared, microwave, radio- and low frequency radiation; coherent radiation produced by stimulated emission; and infrasonic, sonic, and ultrasonic vibrations [281].

There are two main organizations, which are typically issuing international standards, namely, the International Organization for Standardization (ISO) and the International Electrotechnical Commission (IEC). Every region (e.g., EU) or a country (e.g., Japan) has a standard organization that may adopt the established international standards and in some certain cases may modify it or place limitations on it. Furthermore, the local medical device authorities may recognize the standard, but normally there is no legal obligation to do so. In other words, a certain international standard does not define in itself, where it operates. Consequently, any country or region may adopt them, possibly with certain modifications or limitations. For example, in EU, all medical devices, which are intended for use within the EU region, must conform to the Medical Device Directive 93/42/EEC (MDD) [282], which was updated by the Directive 2007-47-EC [283], and must have a CE conformance mark [284].

The following relevant standards are mostly and generally requested (this is not an exhaustive list, and some might not be applicable for the existing solutions, and furthermore, at the same time, some more standards could be relevant):

- ISO 13485:2012 – Medical devices – Quality management systems – Requirements for regulatory purposes. ISO 13485:2012 is applicable only to manufacturers placing devices on the market in Europe. For the rest of the world, the older version ISO 13485:2003 remains the applicable standard [285].

- ISO 14971:2012 – Medical devices – Application of risk management to medical devices [286].
- IEC 60601–1:2015 SER – Medical electrical equipment – All parts [287].
- IECEE TRF 60601-1-2:2015 – Medical electrical equipment – Part 1–2: General requirements for basic safety and essential performance – Collateral standard: Electromagnetic disturbances – Requirements and tests [288].
- IECEE TRF 60601-1-6:2014 – Medical electrical equipment – Part 1–2: General requirements for basic safety and essential performance – Collateral standard: Usability [289].
- IEC 60601-1-8:2006 – Medical electrical equipment – Part 1–8: General requirements for basic safety and essential performance – Collateral standard: General requirements, tests, and guidance for alarm systems in medical electrical equipment and medical electrical systems [290] (included in [287]).
- EN 60601-1-9:2007 – Medical electrical equipment – Part 1–9: General requirements for basic safety and essential performance – Collateral Standard: Requirements for environmentally conscious design [291] (included in [287]).
- IEC 60601-1-11:2015 – Medical electrical equipment – Part 1–11: General requirements for basic safety and essential performance – Collateral standard: Requirements for medical electrical equipment and medical electrical systems used in the home healthcare environment [292] (included in [287]).
- EN 62304:2006 – Medical device software – Software life cycle processes [293].
- ISO 10993:2009 – Biological evaluation of medical devices – Part 1: Evaluation and testing within a risk management process [294].
- ISO 15223–1:2012 – Symbols to be used with medical device labels, labeling, and information to be supplied – Part 1: General requirements [295].
- EN 1041:2008+A1:2013 – Information supplied by the manufacturer of medical devices [296].
- ISO 14155:2011 – Clinical investigation of medical devices for human subjects – Good clinical practice [297].
- MEDDEV 2.7.1 Rev. 3:2009 – Clinical evaluation: A guide for manufacturers and notified bodies [298].
- IEC 62366–1:2015 – Medical devices – Part 1: Application of usability engineering to medical devices [299].
- ISO/IEC 27001 – Information security management [300].
- ISO/IEC 25010:2011 – Systems and software engineering – Systems and software Quality Requirements and Evaluation (SQuaRE) – System and software quality models [301].

The aforementioned standards facilitate so-called harmonized medical device regulatory requirements, and more comprehensive and updated list of titles and references of the harmonized standards under EU harmonization legislation is available on the European Commission web site [302].

As an important note, any software, which is related to the monitoring technology in our context, must also fulfill the aforementioned requirements of the medical device wherein it is incorporated. One can typically divide software in two groups.

First, there is so-called embedded software, which is incorporated in the apparatus, i.e., in a physical device being used for monitoring. Second, there is software that is used in combination with the apparatus but is separate from the device, i.e., software that is involved, for instance, in transferring, receiving, storing, processing, and accessing the data. Both types of software fall under the definition of a "medical device," as we previously mentioned, since it affects the use of the devices. According to the essential requirements of European Medical Device Directive, such software "must be validated according to state of the art taking into account the principles of development lifecycle, risk management, validation and verification" (Annex I, 93/42/EEC as amended by Directive 2007/47/EC [282]). There are numerous specific standards for each area of interest; for example, for the ECG measurement devices, the health informatics standards, such as ISO 11073–91064:2009, ISO/TS 22077–2:2015, and ISO/TS 22077–3:2015, are relevant. Furthermore, in accordance with the current security standards (such as ISO/IEC 27001 [300]), the availability, integrity, and confidentiality of the monitored data and information must be ensured. Last but not least, several generic standards must be followed. For example, ISO/IEC 25010:2011 [301] is necessary for every computer system and software products in general.

In general, most of the national and international standards, for example, those that are published by ISO and IEC, are unfortunately not available free of charge, since there is a certain fee for obtaining them. Furthermore, each individual standard may include many cross-references to other standards. In the field of health telemonitoring, the number of relevant standards is substantially high. Therefore, for many stakeholders this would result in extra investments, which can be increasingly high due to the fact that these standards are frequently updated and manufacturers have to constantly adapt to the state of the art.

As a solution, the responsible authorities for safeguarding the quality and reliability of various health telemonitoring solutions should in principle promote an open access to the relevant standards, or at least help to improve their availability to those who develop and deliver health telemonitoring products and services. This solution is in agreement with previously proposed suggestions [303]. Alternatively, some reimbursement strategies for successful implementation of those standards might be initiated, which could further motivate the compliance with those important standards for further quality improvement of the healthcare.

References

1. Pogorelc, B., Gams, M.: Home-based health monitoring of the elderly through gait recognition. J. Ambient Intell. Smart Environ. **4**(5), 415–428 (2012)
2. Kempe, V.: Inertial MEMS: Principles and Practice, 1st edn. Cambridge University Press, Cambridge/New York (2011)
3. Stone, E., Skubic, M.: Evaluation of an inexpensive depth camera for in-home gait assessment. J. Ambient Intell. Smart Env. **3**(4), 349–361 (2011)

4. Vatavu, R.-D.: Nomadic gestures: a technique for reusing gesture commands for frequent ambient interactions. J. Ambient Intell. Smart Environ. **4**(2), 79–93 (2012)
5. Poppe, R.: Vision-based human motion analysis: an overview. Comput. Vis. Image Underst. **108**(1–2), 4–18 (2007)
6. Matsukawa, T., Umetani, T., Yokoyama, K.: Development of health monitoring system based on three-dimensional imaging using bio-signals and motion data. In: 29th Annual International Conference of the IEEE Engineering in Medicine and Biology Society, 2007. EMBS 2007, pp. 1523–1527 (2007)
7. Kaushik, A., Lovell, N., Celler, B.: Evaluation of PIR detector characteristics for monitoring occupancy patterns of elderly people living alone at home. In: 29th Annual International Conference of the IEEE Engineering in Medicine and Biology Society, 2007. EMBS 2007, pp. 3802–3805 (2007)
8. Miskelly, F.G.: Assistive technology in elderly care. Age Ageing **30**(6), 455–458 (2001)
9. Chen, B.-R., Patel, S., Buckley, T., Rednic, R., McClure, D.J., Shih, L., Tarsy, D., Welsh, M., Bonato, P.: A web-based system for home monitoring of patients with Parkinson's disease using wearable sensors. IEEE Trans. Biomed. Eng. **58**(3), 831–836 (2011)
10. Chiang, C.-Y., Chen, Y.-L., Yu, C.-W., Yuan, S.-M., Hong, Z.-W.: An efficient component-based framework for intelligent home-care system design with video and physiological monitoring machineries. In: 2011 Fifth International Conference on Genetic and Evolutionary Computing (ICGEC), pp. 33–36 (2011)
11. Confidence Consortium: Ubiquitous care system to support independent living. FP7-ICT-214986 (2011)
12. Colizzi, L., Savino, N., Rametta, P., Rizzi, L., Fiorino, G., Piccininno, G., Piccinno, M., Rana, G., Petrosillo, F., Natrella, M., Laneve, L.: H@H: a telemedicine suite for de-hospitalization of chronic disease patients. In: 2010 10th IEEE International Conference on Information Technology and Applications in Biomedicine (ITAB), pp. 1–4 (2010)
13. Lau, C., Churchill, R.S., Kim, J., Matsen, F.A., Kim, Y.: Asynchronous web-based patient-centered home telemedicine system. IEEE Trans. Biomed. Eng. **49**(12), 1452–1462 (2002)
14. Pitta, F., Troosters, T., Spruit, M.A., Decramer, M., Gosselink, R.: Activity monitoring for assessment of physical activities in daily life in patients with chronic obstructive pulmonary disease. Arch. Phys. Med. Rehabil. **86**(10), 1979–1985 (2005)
15. Shoaib, M., Dragon, R., Ostermann, J.: View-invariant fall detection for elderly in real home environment. In: 2010 Fourth Pacific-Rim Symposium on Image and Video Technology (PSIVT), pp. 52–57 (2010)
16. Rougier, C., Meunier, J., St-Arnaud, A., Rousseau, J.: Robust video surveillance for fall detection based on human shape deformation. IEEE Trans. Circuits Syst. Video Technol. **21**(5), 611–622 (2011)
17. Foroughi, H., Rezvanian, A., Paziraee, A.: Robust fall detection using human shape and multi-class support vector machine. In: Sixth Indian Conference on Computer Vision, Graphics Image Processing, 2008. ICVGIP '08, pp. 413–420 (2008)
18. Meffre, A., Collet, C., Lachiche, N., Gançarski, P.: Real-time fall detection method based on hidden Markov modelling. In: Elmoataz, A., Mammass, D., Lezoray, O., Nouboud, F., Aboutajdine, D. (eds.) Image and Signal Processing, pp. 521–530. Springer, Berlin/Heidelberg (2012)
19. Foroughi, H., Aski, B.S., Pourreza, H.: Intelligent video surveillance for monitoring fall detection of elderly in home environments. In: 11th International Conference on Computer and Information Technology, 2008. ICCIT 2008, pp. 219–224 (2008)
20. Yu, X., Wang, X., Kittipanya-Ngam, P., Eng, H.L., Cheong, L.-F.: Fall detection and alert for ageing-at-home of elderly. In: Mokhtari, M., Khalil, I., Bauchet, J., Zhang, D., Nugent, C. (eds.) Ambient Assistive Health and Wellness Management in the Heart of the City, pp. 209–216. Springer, Berlin/Heidelberg (2009)

21. Crispim-Junior, C.F., Bremond, F., Joumier, V.: A multi-sensor approach for activity recognition in older patients. Presented at the Second International Conference on Ambient Computing, Applications, Services and Technologies – AMBIENT 2012 (2012)
22. Zhou, Z., Chen, X., Chung, Y.-C., He, Z., Han, T.X., Keller J.M.: Video-based activity monitoring for indoor environments. In: IEEE International Symposium on Circuits and Systems, 2009. ISCAS 2009, pp. 1449–1452 (2009)
23. Banerjee, T., Keller, J., Skubic, M., Stone, E.: Day or night activity recognition from video using fuzzy clustering techniques. IEEE Trans. Fuzzy Syst. Early Access Online, (2013)
24. Sim, K., Yap, G.-E., Phua, C., Biswas, J., Wai, A.A.P., Tolstikov, A., Huang, W., Yap, P.: Improving the accuracy of erroneous-plan recognition system for activities of daily living. In: 2010 12th IEEE International Conference on e-Health Networking Applications and Services (Healthcom), pp. 28–35 (2010)
25. Pirsiavash, H., Ramanan, D.: Detecting activities of daily living in first-person camera views. In: 2012 IEEE Conference on Computer Vision and Pattern Recognition (CVPR), pp. 2847–2854 (2012)
26. Messing, R., Pal, C., Kautz, H.: Activity recognition using the velocity histories of tracked keypoints. In: 2009 IEEE 12th International Conference on Computer Vision, pp. 104–111 (2009)
27. Schuldt, C., Laptev, I., Caputo, B.: Recognizing human actions: a local SVM approach. In: Proceedings of the 17th International Conference on Pattern Recognition, 2004. ICPR 2004, vol. 3, pp. 32–36 (2004)
28. Ma, Q., Fosty, B., Crispim-Junior, C.F., Bremond, F.: Fusion framework for video event recognition. Presented at the 10th IASTED International Conference on Signal Processing, Pattern Recognition and Applications (2013)
29. Tang, Y., Ma, B., Yan, H.: Intelligent video surveillance system for elderly people living alone based on ODVS. Adv. Internet Things **03**(02), 44–52 (2013)
30. van Kasteren, T.L.M., Englebienne, G., Kröse, B.J.A.: An activity monitoring system for elderly care using generative and discriminative models. Pers. Ubiquit Comput. **14**(6), 489–498 (2010)
31. Hasanuzzaman, F.M., Yang, X., Tian, Y., Liu, Q., Capezuti, E.: Monitoring activity of taking medicine by incorporating RFID and video analysis. Netw. Model. Anal. Health Inform. Bioinforma. **2**(2), 61–70 (2013)
32. Zouba, N., Bremond, F., Thonnat, M.: An activity monitoring system for real elderly at home: validation study. In: 2010 Seventh IEEE International Conference on Advanced Video and Signal Based Surveillance (AVSS), pp. 278–285 (2010)
33. Zhong, H., Shi, J., Visontai, M.: Detecting unusual activity in video. In: Proceedings of the 2004 IEEE Computer Society Conference on Computer Vision and Pattern Recognition, 2004. CVPR 2004, vol. 2, pp. II–819–II–826 (2004)
34. Nait-Charif, H., McKenna, S.J.: Activity summarisation and fall detection in a supportive home environment. In: Proceedings of the 17th International Conference on Pattern Recognition, 2004. ICPR 2004, vol. 4, pp. 323–326 (2004)
35. Lin, C.-W., Ling, Z.-H.: Automatic fall incident detection in compressed video for intelligent homecare. In: Proceedings of 16th International Conference on Computer Communications and Networks, 2007. ICCCN 2007, pp. 1172–1177 (2007)
36. Belshaw, M., Taati, B., Giesbrecht, D., Mihailidis, A.: Intelligent vision-based fall detection system: preliminary results from a real-world deployment. In RESNA/ICTA, Toronto (2011)
37. Poh, M.-Z., McDuff, D.J., Picard, R.W.: Advancements in noncontact, multiparameter physiological measurements using a webcam. IEEE Trans. Biomed. Eng. **58**(1), 7–11 (2011)
38. Kwon, S., Kim, H., Park, K.S.: Validation of heart rate extraction using video imaging on a built-in camera system of a smartphone. In: 2012 Annual International Conference of the IEEE Engineering in Medicine and Biology Society (EMBC), pp. 2174–2177 (2012)

39. Scully, C., Lee, J., Meyer, J., Gorbach, A.M., Granquist-Fraser, D., Mendelson, Y., Chon, K.H.: Physiological parameter monitoring from optical recordings with a mobile phone. IEEE Trans. Biomed. Eng. **59**(2), 303–306 (2012)
40. Kim, B., Lee, S., Cho, D., Oh, S.: A proposal of heart diseases diagnosis method using analysis of face color. In: International Conference on Advanced Language Processing and Web Information Technology, 2008. ALPIT '08, pp. 220–225 (2008)
41. Haque, M.A., Nasrollahi, K., Moeslund, T.B.: Constructing facial expression log from video sequences using face quality assessment. Presented at the International Conference on Computer Vision Theory and Applications, Lisbon (2014)
42. Chen, D., Bharucha, A.J., Wactlar, H.D.: Intelligent video monitoring to improve safety of older persons. In: 29th Annual International Conference of the IEEE Engineering in Medicine and Biology Society, 2007. EMBS 2007, pp. 3814–3817 (2007)
43. Stone, E.E., Skubic, M.: Fall detection in homes of older adults using the Microsoft Kinect. IEEE J. Biomed. Health Inform. **19**(1), 290–301 (2015)
44. Spinsante, S., Antonicelli, R., Mazzanti, I., Gambi, E.: Technological approaches to remote monitoring of elderly people in cardiology: a usability perspective. Int. J. Telemed. Appl. (2012). doi:10.1155/2012/104561
45. Salleh, S.H., Hussain, H.S., Swee, T.T., Ting, C.-M., Noor, A.M., Pipatsart, S., Ali, J., Yupapin, P.P.: Acoustic cardiac signals analysis: a Kalman filter-based approach. Int. J. Nanomedicine **7**, 2873–2881 (2012)
46. Emmanuel, B.S.: A review of signal processing techniques for heart sound analysis in clinical diagnosis. J. Med. Eng. Technol. **36**(6), 303–307 (2012)
47. Tsanas, A., Little, M.A., McSharry, P.E., Spielman, J., Ramig, L.O.: Novel speech signal processing algorithms for high-accuracy classification of Parkinson's disease. IEEE Trans. Biomed. Eng. **59**(5), 1264–1271 (2012)
48. Ng, A.K., Koh, T.-S.: Using psychoacoustics of snoring sounds to screen for obstructive sleep apnea. In: 30th Annual International Conference of the IEEE Engineering in Medicine and Biology Society, 2008. EMBS 2008, pp. 1647–1650 (2008)
49. Vacher, M., Fleury, A., Portet, F., Serignat, J.-F., Noury, N.: Complete sound and speech recognition system for health smart homes: application to the recognition of activities of daily living. In: Campolo, D. (ed.) New Developments in Biomedical Engineering. InTech, Rijeka (2010)
50. Ye, J., Kobayashi, T., Higuchi, T.: Audio-based indoor health monitoring system using FLAC features. In: 2010 International Conference on Emerging Security Technologies (EST), pp. 90–95 (2010)
51. Kepski, M., Kwolek, B.: Human fall detection using kinect sensor. In: Burduk, R., Jackowski, K., Kurzynski, M., Wozniak, M., Zolnierek, A. (eds.) Proceedings of the 8th International Conference on Computer Recognition Systems CORES 2013, pp. 743–752. Springer, Heidelberg (2013)
52. Charlon, Y., Bourennane, W., Bettahar, F., Campo, E.: Activity monitoring system for elderly in a context of smart home. IRBM **34**(1), 60–63 (2013)
53. Naranjo-Hernandez, D., Roa, L.M., Reina-Tosina, J., Estudillo-Valderrama, M.A.: SoM: a smart sensor for human activity monitoring and assisted healthy ageing. IEEE Trans. Biomed. Eng. **59**(11), 3177–3184 (2012)
54. Bourke, A.K., Scanaill, C.N., Culhane, K.M., O'Brien, J.V., Lyons, G.M.: An optimum accelerometer configuration and simple algorithm for accurately detecting falls. In: Proceedings of the 24th IASTED International Conference on Biomedical Engineering, pp. 156–160. Anaheim (2006)
55. Yuwono, M., Moulton, B.D., Su, S.W., Celler, B.G., Nguyen, H.T.: Unsupervised machine-learning method for improving the performance of ambulatory fall-detection systems. Biomed. Eng. Online **11**(1), 9 (2012)
56. Kurella Tamura, M., Covinsky, K.E., Chertow, G.M., Yaffe, K., Landefeld, C.S., McCulloch, C.E.: Functional status of elderly adults before and after initiation of dialysis. N. Engl. J. Med. **361**(16), 1539–1547 (2009)

57. Silva, M., Teixeira, P.M., Abrantes, F., Sousa, F.: Design and evaluation of a fall detection algorithm on mobile phone platform. In: Gabrielli, S., Elias, D., Kahol, K. (eds.) Ambient Media and Systems, pp. 28–35. Springer, Berlin/Heidelberg (2011)
58. Tong, L., Song, Q., Ge, Y., Liu, M.: HMM-based human fall detection and prediction method using tri-axial accelerometer. IEEE Sens. J. **13**(5), 1849–1856 (2013)
59. Zhang, T., Wang, J., Xu, L., Liu, P.: Fall detection by wearable sensor and one-class SVM algorithm. In: Huang, D.-S., Li, K., Irwin, G.W. (eds.) Intelligent Computing in Signal Processing and Pattern Recognition, pp. 858–863. Springer, Berlin/Heidelberg (2006)
60. Alam, M.A., Wang, W., Ahamed, S.I., Chu, W.: Elderly safety: a smartphone based real time approach. In: Biswas, J., Kobayashi, H., Wong, L., Abdulrazak, B., Mokhtari, M. (eds.) Inclusive Society: Health and Wellbeing in the Community, and Care at Home, pp. 134–142. Springer, Berlin/Heidelberg (2013)
61. Sasidhar, S., Panda, S.K., Xu, J.: A wavelet feature based mechanomyography classification system for a wearable rehabilitation system for the elderly. In: Biswas, J., Kobayashi, H., Wong, L., Abdulrazak, B., Mokhtari, M. (eds.) Inclusive Society: Health and Wellbeing in the Community, and Care at Home, pp. 45–52. Springer, Berlin/Heidelberg (2013)
62. Chen, G.-C., Huang, C.-N., Chiang, C.-Y., Hsieh, C.-J., Chan, C.-T.: A reliable fall detection system based on wearable sensor and signal magnitude area for elderly residents. In: Lee, Y., Bien, Z.Z., Mokhtari, M., Kim, J.T., Park, M., Kim, J., Lee, H., Khalil, I. (eds.) Aging Friendly Technology for Health and Independence, pp. 267–270. Springer, Berlin/Heidelberg (2010)
63. Yu, F., Bilberg, A., Stenager, E., Rabotti, C., Zhang, B., Mischi, M.: A wireless body measurement system to study fatigue in multiple sclerosis. Physiol. Meas. **33**(12), 2033 (2012)
64. Dobkin, B.H., Dorsch, A.: The promise of mHealth daily activity monitoring and outcome assessments by wearable sensors. Neurorehabil. Neural Repair **25**(9), 788–798 (2011)
65. Luštrek, M., Kaluža, B.: Fall detection and activity recognition with machine learning. Informatica **33**, 205–212 (2009)
66. Pogorelc, B., Bosnić, Z., Gams, M.: Automatic recognition of gait-related health problems in the elderly using machine learning. Multimed. Tools Appl. **58**(2), 333–354 (2012)
67. Zhou, M., Wang, S., Chen, Y., Chen, Z., Zhao, Z.: An activity transition based fall detection model on mobile devices. In: Park, J.H.J., Jin, Q., Yeo, M.S., Hu, B. (eds.) Human Centric Technology and Service in Smart Space, pp. 1–8. Springer, Netherlands (2012)
68. Remoortel, H.V., Giavedoni, S., Raste, Y., Burtin, C., Louvaris, Z., Gimeno-Santos, E., Langer, D., Glendenning, A., Hopkinson, N.S., Vogiatzis, I., Peterson, B.T., Wilson, F., Mann, B., Rabinovich, R., Puhan, M.A., Troosters, T.: Validity of activity monitors in health and chronic disease: a systematic review. Int. J. Behav. Nutr. Phys. Act. **9**(1), 84 (2012)
69. Silva, B.M.C., Rodrigues, J.J.P.C., Simoes, T.M.C., Sendra, S., Lloret, J.: An ambient assisted living framework for mobile environments. In: 2014 IEEE-EMBS International Conference on Biomedical and Health Informatics (BHI), pp. 448–451 (2014)
70. Monte-Moreno, E.: Non-invasive estimate of blood glucose and blood pressure from a photoplethysmograph by means of machine learning techniques. Artif. Intell. Med. **53**(2), 127–138 (2011)
71. Mann, W.C., Marchant, T., Tomita, M., Fraas, L., Stanton, K.: Elder acceptance of health monitoring devices in the home. Care Manag. J. J. Case Manag. J. Long Term Home Health Care **3**(2), 91–98 (2001/2002)
72. Qiu, C., Winblad, B., Fratiglioni, L.: The age-dependent relation of blood pressure to cognitive function and dementia. Lancet Neurol. **4**(8), 487–499 (2005)
73. Fagard, R.H., Van Den Broeke, C., De Cort, P.: Prognostic significance of blood pressure measured in the office, at home and during ambulatory monitoring in older patients in general practice. J. Hum. Hypertens. **19**(10), 801–807 (2005)
74. Ilie, B.: Portable equipment for monitoring human functional parameters. In: 9th Roedunet International Conference (RoEduNet), 2010, pp. 299–302 (2010)
75. Brindel, P., Hanon, O., Dartigues, J.-F., Ritchie, K., Lacombe, J.-M., Ducimetiere, P., Alperovitch, A., Tzourio, C., 3C Study Investigators: Prevalence, awareness, treatment, and control of hypertension in the elderly: the three city study. J. Hypertens. **24**(1), 51–58 (2006). January 2006

76. Nishida, Y., Hori, T.: Non-invasive and unrestrained monitoring of human respiratory system by sensorized environment. In: Proceedings of IEEE Sensors, 2002, vol. 1, pp. 705–710 (2002)
77. Lee, H., Kim, Y.T., Jung, J.W., Park, K.H., Kim, D.J., Bang, B., Bien, Z.Z.: A 24-hour health monitoring system in a smart house. Gerontechnology **7**(1), 22–35 (2008)
78. Fiedler, P., Biller, S., Griebel, S., Haueisen, J.: Impedance pneumography using textile electrodes. In: 2012 Annual International Conference of the IEEE Engineering in Medicine and Biology Society (EMBC), pp. 1606–1609 (2012)
79. Chaudhry, S.I., Mattera, J.A., Curtis, J.P., Spertus, J.A., Herrin, J., Lin, Z., Phillips, C.O., Hodshon, B.V., Cooper, L.S., Krumholz, H.M.: Telemonitoring in patients with heart failure. N. Engl. J. Med. **363**(24), 2301–2309 (2010)
80. Raad, M.W., Yang, L.T.: A ubiquitous smart home for elderly. In: 4th IET International Conference on Advances in Medical, Signal and Information Processing, 2008. MEDSIP 2008, pp. 1–4 (2008)
81. Chung, W.-Y., Bhardwaj, S., Punvar, A., Lee, D.-S., Myllylae, R.: A fusion health monitoring using ECG and accelerometer sensors for elderly persons at home. In: Annual International Conference IEEE Engineering in Medical and Biology Society, vol. 2007, pp. 3818–3821 (2007)
82. Chi, Y.M., Cauwenberghs, G.: Wireless non-contact EEG/ECG electrodes for body sensor networks. In: 2010 International Conference on Body Sensor Networks (BSN), pp. 297–301 (2010)
83. Chi, Y.M., Deiss, S.R., Cauwenberghs, G.: Non-contact low power EEG/ECG electrode for high density wearable biopotential sensor networks. In: Sixth International Workshop on Wearable and Implantable Body Sensor Networks, 2009. BSN 2009, pp. 246–250 (2009)
84. Snogdal, L.S., Folkestad, L., Elsborg, R., Remvig, L.S., Beck-Nielsen, H., Thorsteinsson, B., Jennum, P., Gjerstad, M., Juhl, C.B.: Detection of hypoglycemia associated EEG changes during sleep in type 1 diabetes mellitus. Diabetes Res. Clin. Pract. **98**(1), 91–97 (2012)
85. Chi, Y.M., Ng, P., Kang, E., Kang, J., Fang, J., Cauwenberghs, G.: Wireless non-contact cardiac and neural monitoring. In: Wireless Health 2010, pp. 15–23. ACM, New York (2010)
86. Klonovs, J., Petersen, C.K., Olesen, H., Hammershoj, A.: ID proof on the go: development of a mobile EEG-based biometric authentication system. IEEE Veh. Technol. Mag. **8**(1), 81–89 (2013)
87. Henderson, G., Ifeachor, E., Hudson, N., Goh, C., Outram, N., Wimalaratna, S., Del Percio, C., Vecchio, F.: Development and assessment of methods for detecting dementia using the human electroencephalogram. IEEE Trans. Biomed. Eng. **53**(8), 1557–1568 (2006)
88. Nguyen, H.T., Jones, T.W.: Detection of nocturnal hypoglycemic episodes using EEG signals. In: 2010 Annual International Conference of the IEEE Engineering in Medicine and Biology Society (EMBC), pp. 4930–4933 (2010)
89. Abdullah, H., Maddage, N.C., Cosic, I., Cvetkovic, D.: Cross-correlation of EEG frequency bands and heart rate variability for sleep apnoea classification. Med. Biol. Eng. Comput. **48**(12), 1261–1269 (2010)
90. Juhl, C.B., Højlund, K., Elsborg, R., Poulsen, M.K., Selmar, P.E., Holst, J.J., Christiansen, C., Beck-Nielsen, H.: Automated detection of hypoglycemia-induced EEG changes recorded by subcutaneous electrodes in subjects with type 1 diabetes – the brain as a biosensor. Diabetes Res. Clin. Pract. **88**(1), 22–28 (2010)
91. Harikumar, R., Ganeshbabu, C., Balasubramani, M., Sinthiya, P.: Analysis of SVD neural networks for classification of epilepsy risk level from EEG signals. In: Mohan. S., Kumar, S.S. (eds.) Proceedings of the Fourth International Conference on Signal and Image Processing 2012 (ICSIP 2012), pp. 27–34. Springer, India (2013)
92. Martín-Lesende, I., Orruño, E., Bilbao, A., Vergara, I., Cairo, M.C., Bayón, J.C., Reviriego, E., Romo, M.I., Larrañaga, J., Asua, J., Abad, R., Recalde, E.: Impact of telemonitoring home care patients with heart failure or chronic lung disease from primary care on healthcare resource use (the TELBIL study randomised controlled trial). BMC Health Serv. Res. **13**(1), 118 (2013)

93. Segrelles Calvo, G., Gómez-Suárez, C., Soriano, J.B., Zamora, E., Gónzalez-Gamarra, A., González-Béjar, M., Jordán, A., Tadeo, E., Sebastián, A., Fernández, G., Ancochea, J.: A home telehealth program for patients with severe COPD: the PROMETE study. Respir. Med. **108**(3), 453–462 (2014)
94. Palumbo, F., Ullberg, J., Štimec, A., Furfari, F., Karlsson, L., Coradeschi, S.: Sensor network infrastructure for a home care monitoring system. Sensors **14**(3), 3833–3860 (2014)
95. Keenan, D.B., Mastrototaro, J.J., Voskanyan, G., Steil, G.M.: Delays in minimally invasive continuous glucose monitoring devices: a review of current technology. J. Diabetes Sci. Technol. **3**(5), 1207–1214 (2009)
96. Rowe, M., Lane, S., Phipps, C.: Care watch: a home monitoring system for use in homes of persons with cognitive impairment. Top. Geriatr. Rehabil. **23**(1), 3–8 (2007)
97. Seelye, A.M., Schmitter-Edgecombe, M., Cook, D.J., Crandall, A.: Naturalistic assessment of everyday activities and prompting technologies in mild cognitive impairment. J. Int. Neuropsychol. Soc. **19**(04), 442–452 (2013)
98. Smith, J.R., Fishkin, K.P., Jiang, B., Mamishev, A., Philipose, M., Rea, A.D., Roy, S., Sundara-Rajan, K.: RFID-based techniques for human-activity detection. Commun. ACM **48**(9), 39–44 (2005)
99. Cislo, N.: Undernutrition prevention for disabled and elderly people in smart home with Bayesian networks and RFID sensors. In: Lee, Y., Bien, Z.Z., Mokhtari, M., Kim, J.T., Park, M., Kim, J., Lee, H., Khalil, I. (eds.) Aging Friendly Technology for Health and Independence, pp. 246–249. Springer, Berlin/Heidelberg (2010)
100. Kim, S.-C., Jeong, Y.-S., Park, S.-O.: RFID-based indoor location tracking to ensure the safety of the elderly in smart home environments. Pers. Ubiquitous Comput. **17**(8), 1699–1707 (2013)
101. Mateska, A., Pavloski, M., Gavrilovska, L.: RFID and sensors enabled in-home elderly care. In: 2011 Proceedings of the 34th International Convention MIPRO, pp. 285–290 (2011)
102. Pérez, M.M., Cabrero-Canosa, M., Hermida, J.V., García, L.C., Gómez, D.L., González, G.V., Herranz, I.M.: Application of RFID technology in patient tracking and medication traceability in emergency care. J. Med. Syst. **36**(6), 3983–3993 (2012)
103. Sum, K.W., Zheng, Y.P., Mak, A.F.T.: Vital sign monitoring for elderly at home: development of a compound sensor for pulse rate and motion. Stud. Health Technol. Inform. **117**, 43–50 (2005)
104. Fleury, A., Vacher, M., Noury, N., Member, S.: SVM-based multimodal classification of activities of daily living in health smart homes: Sensors, algorithms, and first experimental results. IEEE Trans. Inf. Technol. Biomed. **14**, 274–283 (2010)
105. Chiriac, S., Saurer, B.R., Stummer, G., Kunze, C.: Introducing a low-cost ambient monitoring system for activity recognition. In: 2011 5th International Conference on Pervasive Computing Technologies for Healthcare (PervasiveHealth), pp. 340–345 (2011)
106. Franco, C., Diot, B., Fleury, A., Demongeot, J., Vuillerme, N.: Ambient assistive healthcare and wellness management – is 'the wisdom of the body' transposable to one's home? In: Biswas, J., Kobayashi, H., Wong, L., Abdulrazak, B., Mokhtari, M. (eds.) Inclusive Society: Health and Wellbeing in the Community, and Care at Home, pp. 143–150. Springer, Berlin/Heidelberg (2013)
107. Suryadevara, N.K., Gaddam, A., Rayudu, R.K., Mukhopadhyay, S.C.: Wireless sensors network based safe home to care elderly people: behaviour detection. Sens. Actuators Phys. **186**, 277–283 (2012)
108. Pogorelc, B., Gams, M.: Discovering the chances of health problems and falls in the elderly using data mining. In: Ohsawa, Y., Abe, A. (eds.) Advances in Chance Discovery, pp. 163–175. Springer, Berlin/Heidelberg (2013)
109. Kaluža, B., Mirchevska, V., Dovgan, E., Luštrek, M., Gams, M.: An agent-based approach to care in independent living. In: de Ruyter, B., Wichert, R., Keyson, D.V., Markopoulos, P., Streitz, N., Divitini, M., Georgantas, N., Gomez, A.M. (eds.) Ambient Intelligence, pp. 177–186. Springer, Berlin/Heidelberg (2010)

110. Kaluža, B., Gams, M.: Analysis of daily-living dynamics. J. Ambient Intell. Smart Environ. **4**(5), 403–413 (2012)
111. Yu, X.: Approaches and principles of fall detection for elderly and patient, In: 10th International Conference on e-health Networking, Applications and Services, 2008. HealthCom 2008, pp. 42–47 (2008)
112. Wang, X., Li, M., Ji, H., Gong, Z.: A novel modeling approach to fall detection and experimental validation using motion capture system. In: 2013 IEEE International Conference on Robotics and Biomimetics (ROBIO), pp. 234–239 (2013)
113. Cheng, L., Shum, V., Kuntze, G., McPhillips, G., Wilson, A., Hailes, S., Kerwin, D., Kerwin, G.: A wearable and flexible bracelet computer for on-body sensing. In: 2011 IEEE Consumer Communications and Networking Conference (CCNC), pp. 860–864 (2011)
114. British Standards: BS 8300:2009+A1:2010 Design of buildings and their approaches to meet the needs of disabled people. 28 Feb 2009
115. International Organization for Standardization: ISO 21542:2011: building construction – accessibility and usability of the built environment (2011)
116. Austin, D., Hayes, T.L., Kaye, J., Mattek, N., Pavel, M.: Unobtrusive monitoring of the longitudinal evolution of in-home gait velocity data with applications to elder care. In: Conference Proceedings Annual International Conference of IEEE Engineering in Medical and Biology Society, vol. 2011, pp. 6495–6498 (2011)
117. Kaushik, A.R., Lovell, N.H., Celler, B.G.: Evaluation of PIR detector characteristics for monitoring occupancy patterns of elderly people living alone at home. In: Conference Proceedings Annual International Conference of IEEE Engineering in Medical and Biology Society, vol. 2007, pp. 3802–3805 (2007)
118. Kaushik, A.R., Lovell, N.H., Celler, B.G.: Evaluation of PIR detector characteristics for monitoring occupancy patterns of elderly people living alone at home. In: 29th Annual International Conference of the IEEE Engineering in Medicine and Biology Society, 2007. EMBS 2007, pp. 3802–3805 (2007)
119. Kaushik, A.R., Celler, B.G.: Characterization of PIR detector for monitoring occupancy patterns and functional health status of elderly people living alone at home. Technol. Health Care **15**(4), 273–288 (2007)
120. Franco, C., Demongeot, J., Villemazet, C., Vuillerme, N.: Behavioral telemonitoring of the elderly at home: detection of nycthemeral rhythms drifts from location data. In: 2010 IEEE 24th International Conference on Advanced Information Networking and Applications Workshops (WAINA), pp. 759–766 (2010)
121. Panek, P., Mayer, P.: Monitoring system for day-to-day activities of older persons living at home alone. Gerontechnology **11**(2), 302 (2012)
122. Fei, J., Pavlidis, I.: Thermistor at a distance: unobtrusive measurement of breathing. IEEE Trans. Biomed. Eng. **57**(4), 988–998 (2010)
123. Wolff, L.B., Socolinsky, D.A., Eveland, C.K.: Quantitative Measurement of Illumination Invariance for Face Recognition Using Thermal Infrared Imagery, pp. 140–151 (2003)
124. Stel, V.S., Pluijm, S.M.F., Deeg, D.J.H., Smit, J.H., Bouter, L.M., Lips, P.: A classification tree for predicting recurrent falling in community-dwelling older persons. J. Am. Geriatr. Soc. **51**(10), 1356–1364 (2003)
125. Woolrych, R., Sixsmith, A., Mortenson, B., Robinovitch, S., Feldman, F.: The nature and use of surveillance technologies in residential care. In: Biswas, J., Kobayashi, H., Wong, L., Abdulrazak, B., Mokhtari, M. (eds.) Inclusive Society: Health and Wellbeing in the Community, and Care at Home, pp. 1–9. Springer, Berlin/Heidelberg (2013)
126. Ahad, M.A.R., Tan, J., Kim, H., Ishikawa, S.: Action dataset – a survey. In: 2011 Proceedings of SICE Annual Conference (SICE), pp. 1650–1655 (2011)
127. Dikmen, O., Mesaros, A.: Sound event detection using non-negative dictionaries learned from annotated overlapping events. In: 2013 IEEE Workshop on Applications of Signal Processing to Audio and Acoustics (WASPAA), pp. 1–4 (2013)
128. Mesaros, A., Heittola, T., Eronen, A., Virtanen, T.: Acoustic event detection in real life recordings. In: 18th European Signal Processing Conference, pp. 1267–1271 (2010)

129. Vuegen, L., Broeck, B.V.D., Karsmakers, P., Hamme, H.V., Vanrumste, B.: Automatic monitoring of activities of daily living based on real-life acoustic sensor data: a~preliminary study. In: Proceedings Fourth Workshop Speech Language Processing Assistive Technologies, pp. 113–118 (2013)
130. Arlotto, P., Grimaldi, M., Naeck, R., Ginoux, J.-M.: An ultrasonic contactless sensor for breathing monitoring. Sensors **14**(8), 15371–15386 (2014)
131. Lorussi, F., Galatolo, S., De Rossi, D.E.: Textile-based electrogoniometers for wearable posture and gesture capture systems. IEEE Sens. J. **9**(9), 1014–1024 (2009)
132. Carvalho, H., Catarino, A.P., Rocha, A., Postolache, O.: Health monitoring using textile sensors and electrodes: an overview and integration of technologies. In: 2014 IEEE International Symposium on Medical Measurements and Applications (MeMeA), pp. 1–6 (2014)
133. Pacelli, M., Caldani, L., Paradiso, R.: Textile piezoresistive sensors for biomechanical variables monitoring. In: 28th Annual International Conference of the IEEE Engineering in Medicine and Biology Society, 2006. EMBS '06, pp. 5358–5361 (2006)
134. Lee, R.Y.W., Carlisle, A.J.: Detection of falls using accelerometers and mobile phone technology. Age Ageing **40**, 690–696 (2011)
135. Lu, W., Qin, X., Asiri, A.M., Al-Youbi, A.O., Sun, X.: Ni foam: a novel three-dimensional porous sensing platform for sensitive and selective nonenzymatic glucose detection. Analyst **138**(2), 417–420 (2012)
136. Bellazzi, R., Magni, P., De Nicolao, G.: Bayesian analysis of blood glucose time series from diabetes home monitoring. IEEE Trans. Biomed. Eng. **47**(7), 971–975 (2000)
137. Tian, F.C., Kadri, C., Zhang, L., Feng, J.W., Juan, L.H., Na, P.L.: A novel cost-effective portable electronic nose for indoor-/in-car air quality monitoring. In: 2012 International Conference on Computer Distributed Control and Intelligent Environmental Monitoring (CDCIEM), pp. 4–8 (2012)
138. Fonollosa, J., Rodriguez-Lujan, I., Shevade, A.V., Homer, M.L., Ryan, M.A., Huerta, R.: Human activity monitoring using gas sensor arrays. Sens. Actuators B Chem. **199**, 398–402 (2014)
139. Coyle, S., Morris, D., Lau, K.-T., Diamond, D., Di Francesco, F., Taccini, N., Trivella, M. G., Costanzo, D., Salvo, P., Porchet, J.-A., Luprano, J.: Textile sensors to measure sweat pH and sweat-rate during exercise. In: 3rd International Conference on Pervasive Computing Technologies for Healthcare, 2009. PervasiveHealth 2009, pp. 1–6 (2009)
140. Mendes, P.M., Figueiredo, C.P., Fernandes, M., Gama, Ó.S.: Electronics in medicine. In: Kramme, R., Hoffmann, K.-P., Pozos, R.S. (eds.) Springer Handbook of Medical Technology, pp. 1337–1376. Springer, Berlin/Heidelberg (2011)
141. Haahr, R.G., Duun, S., Thomsen, E.V., Hoppe, K., Branebjerg, J.: A wearable 'electronic patch' for wireless continuous monitoring of chronically diseased patients. In: 5th International Summer School and Symposium on Medical Devices and Biosensors, 2008. ISSS-MDBS 2008, pp. 66–70 (2008)
142. Nielsen, D.B., Egstrup, K., Branebjerg, J., Andersen, G.B., Sorensen, H.B.D.: Automatic QRS complex detection algorithm designed for a novel wearable, wireless electrocardiogram recording device. In: 2012 Annual International Conference of the IEEE Engineering in Medicine and Biology Society (EMBC), pp. 2913–2916 (2012)
143. Chernbumroong, S., Cang, S., Atkins, A., Yu, H.: Elderly activities recognition and classification for applications in assisted living. Expert Syst. Appl. **40**(5), 1662–1674 (2013)
144. Demongeot, J., Virone, G., Duchêne, F., Benchetrit, G., Hervé, T., Noury, N., Rialle, V.: Multi-sensors acquisition, data fusion, knowledge mining and alarm triggering in health smart homes for elderly people. C. R. Biol. **325**(6), 673–682 (2002)
145. Rajendran, P., Corcoran, A., Kinosian, B., Alwan, M.: Falls, fall prevention, and fall detection technologies. In: Alwan, M., Felder, R.A. (eds.) Eldercare Technology for Clinical Practitioners, pp. 187–202. Humana Press, Totowa (2008)
146. Degen, T., Jaeckel, H., Rufer, M., Wyss S.: SPEEDY: a fall detector in a wrist watch. In: Proceedings, Seventh IEEE International Symposium on Wearable Computers, 2003, pp. 184–187 (2003)

147. Koenig, S.M., Mack, D., Alwan, M.: Sleep and sleep assessment technologies. In: Alwan, M., Felder, R.A. (eds.) Eldercare Technology for Clinical Practitioners, pp. 77–120. Humana Press, Totowa (2008)
148. Hung, K., Zhang, Y.T., Tai, B.: Wearable medical devices for tele-home healthcare. In: 26th Annual International Conference of the IEEE Engineering in Medicine and Biology Society, 2004. IEMBS '04, vol. 2, pp. 5384–5387 (2004)
149. Sim, S.Y., Jeon, H.S., Chung, G.S., Kim, S.K., Kwon, S.J., Lee, W.K., Park, K.S.: Fall detection algorithm for the elderly using acceleration sensors on the shoes. In: 2011 Annual International Conference of the IEEE Engineering in Medicine and Biology Society, EMBC, pp. 4935–4938 (2011)
150. Lanata, A., Scilingo, E.P., Francesconi, R., Varone, G., De Rossi, D.: New ultrasound-based wearable system for cardiac monitoring. In: 5th IEEE Conference on Sensors, 2006, pp. 489–492 (2006)
151. Dittmar, A., Meffre, R., De Oliveira, F., Gehin C., Delhomme, G.: Wearable medical devices using textile and flexible technologies for ambulatory monitoring. In: 27th Annual International Conference of the Engineering in Medicine and Biology Society, 2005. IEEE-EMBS 2005. pp. 7161–7164 (2005)
152. Megalingam, R.K., Radhakrishnan, V., Jacob, D.C., Unnikrishnan, D.K.M., Sudhakaran, A.K.: Assistive technology for elders: wireless intelligent healthcare gadget. In: 2011 IEEE Global Humanitarian Technology Conference (GHTC), pp. 296–300 (2011)
153. Mohan, A., Devasahayam, S.R., Tharion, G., George, J.: A sensorized glove and ball for monitoring hand rehabilitation therapy in stroke patients. In: India Educators' Conference (TIIEC), 2013 Texas Instruments, pp. 321–327 (2013)
154. Wai, A.A.P., Foo, S.F., Jayachandran, M., Biswas, J., Nugent, C., Mulvenna, M., Zhang, D., Craig, D., Passmore, P., Lee, J.-E., Yap, P.: Towards developing effective Continence Management through wetness alert diaper: experiences, lessons learned, challenges and future directions. In: Pervasive Computing Technologies for Healthcare (PervasiveHealth), 2010 4th International Conference on-NO PERMISSIONS, pp. 1–8 (2010)
155. Rehman, A., Mustafa, M., Javaid, N., Qasim, U., Khan, Z.A.: Analytical survey of wearable sensors, arXiv:1208.2376 (2012)
156. Falk, T.H., Guirgis, M., Power, S., Chau, T.T.: Taking NIRS-BCIs outside the lab: towards achieving robustness against environment noise. IEEE Trans. Neural Syst. Rehabil. Eng. **19**(2), 136–146 (2011)
157. Noury, N., Virone, G., Creuzet, T.: The health integrated smart home information system (HIS2): rules based system for the localization of a human. In: Microtechnologies in Medicine and Biology 2nd Annual International IEEE-EMB Special Topic Conference on, pp. 318–321 (2002)
158. Garbey, M., Sun, N., Merla, A., Pavlidis, I.: Contact-free measurement of cardiac pulse based on the analysis of thermal imagery. IEEE Trans. Biomed. Eng. **54**(8), 1418–1426 (2007)
159. Cheng, R., Heinzelman, W., Sturge-Apple, M., Ignjatovic, Z.: A motion-tracking ultrasonic sensor array for behavioral monitoring. IEEE Sens. J **PP**(99), 1 (2011)
160. Pogorelc, B., Gams, M.: Detecting gait-related health problems of the elderly using multidimensional dynamic time warping approach with semantic attributes. Multimed. Tools Appl. **66**(1), 95–114 (2013)
161. Leser, R., Schleindlhuber, A., Lyons, K., Baca, A.: Accuracy of an UWB-based position tracking system used for time-motion analyses in game sports. Eur. J. Sport Sci. **14**(7), 635–642 (2014)
162. Dovgan, E., Luštrek, M., Pogorelc, B., Gradišek, A., Bruger, H., Gams, M.: Intelligent elderly-care prototype for fall and disease detection. Slov. Med. J **80**(11), 824–831 (2011)
163. Klack, L., Möllering, C., Ziefle, M., Schmitz-Rode, T.: Future care floor: a sensitive floor for movement monitoring and fall detection in home environments. In: Lin, J.C., Nikita, K.S. (eds.) Wireless Mobile Communication and Healthcare, pp. 211–218. Springer, Berlin/Heidelberg (2011)

164. Riley, P.O., Paylo, K.W., Kerrigan, D.C.: Mobility and gait assessment technologies. In: Alwan, M., Felder, R.A. (eds.) Eldercare Technology for Clinical Practitioners, pp. 33–51. Humana Press, Totowa (2008)
165. Ni, H., Abdulrazak, B., Zhang, D., Wu, S.: Unobtrusive sleep posture detection for elder-care in smart home. In: Lee, Y., Bien, Z.Z., Mokhtari, M., Kim, J.T., Park, M., Kim, J., Lee, H., Khalil, I. (eds.) Aging Friendly Technology for Health and Independence, pp. 67–75. Springer, Berlin/Heidelberg (2010)
166. Mutlu, B., Krause, A., Forlizzi, J., Guestrin, C., Hodgins, J.: Robust, low-cost, non-intrusive sensing and recognition of seated postures. In: Proceedings of the 20th Annual ACM Symposium on User Interface Software and Technology, pp. 149–158. New York (2007)
167. Townsend, D.I., Goubran, R., Frize, M., Knoefel, F.: Preliminary results on the effect of sensor position on unobtrusive rollover detection for sleep monitoring in smart homes. In: Annual International Conference of the IEEE Engineering in Medicine and Biology Society, 2009. EMBC 2009, pp. 6135–6138 (2009)
168. Arcelus, A., Veledar, I., Goubran, R., Knoefel, F., Sveistrup, H., Bilodeau, M.: Measurements of sit-to-stand timing and symmetry from bed pressure sensors. IEEE Trans. Instrum. Meas. **60**(5), 1732–1740 (2011)
169. Alwis, L., Sun, T., Grattan, K.T.V.: Optical fibre-based sensor technology for humidity and moisture measurement: review of recent progress. Measurement **46**(10), 4052–4074 (2013)
170. Alwan, M., Rajendran, P.J., Kell, S., Mack, D., Dalal, S., Wolfe, M., Felder, R.: A smart and passive floor-vibration based fall detector for elderly. In: Information and Communication Technologies, 2006. ICTTA '06. 2nd, vol. 1, pp. 1003–1007 (2006)
171. Salvosa, C.B., Payne, P.R., Wheeler, E.F.: Environmental conditions and body temperatures of elderly women living alone or in local authority home. Br. Med. J. **4**(5788), 656–659 (1971)
172. Fleury, A., Noury, N., Vacher, M., Glasson, H., Seri, J.-F.: Sound and speech detection and classification in a health smart home. In: 30th Annual International Conference of the IEEE Engineering in Medicine and Biology Society, 2008. EMBS 2008, pp. 4644–4647 (2008)
173. Virone, G., Istrate, D., Vacher, M., Noury, N., Serignat, J.-F., Demongeot, J.: First steps in data fusion between a multichannel audio acquisition and an information system for home healthcare. In: Proceedings of the 25th Annual International Conference of the IEEE Engineering in Medicine and Biology Society, 2003, vol. 2, pp. 1364–1367 (2003)
174. Solbiati M., Sheldon, R.S.: Implantable rhythm devices in the management of vasovagal syncope. Auton. Neurosci. **184**, 33–39 (2014)
175. Rao, S.S., Paulson, J.A., Saad, R.J., McCallum, R., Parkman, H.P., Kuo, B., Semler, J., Chey, W.D.: 950 assessment of colonic, whole gut and regional transit in elderly constipated and healthy subjects with a novel wireless pH/pressure capsule (SmartPill®). Gastroenterology **136**(5), A–144 (2009)
176. Budinger, T.F.: Biomonitoring with wireless communications. Annu. Rev. Biomed. Eng. **5**(1), 383–412 (2003)
177. Abdulrazak, B., Malik, Y., Arab, F., Reid, S.: Phonage: adapted smartphone for aging population. In: Biswas, J., Kobayashi, H., Wong, L., Abdulrazak, B., Mokhtari, M. (eds.) Inclusive Society: Health and Wellbeing in the Community, and Care at Home, pp. 27–35. Springer, Berlin/Heidelberg (2013)
178. Daytime monitoring of patients with epileptic seizures using a smartphone processing framework and on-body sensors. http://www.tue.nl/publicatie/ep/p/d/ep-uid/280415/. Accessed 16 Aug 2013
179. Ogawa, H., Yonezawa, Y., Maki, H., Sato, H., Caldwell, W.M.: A mobile phone-based safety support system for wandering elderly persons. In: 26th Annual International Conference of the IEEE Engineering in Medicine and Biology Society, 2004. IEMBS '04, vol. 2, pp. 3316–3317 (2004)

180. Coradeschi, S., Cesta, A., Cortellessa, G., Coraci, L., Galindo, C., Gonzalez, J., Karlsson, L., Forsberg, A., Frennert, S., Furfari, F., Loutfi, A., Orlandini, A., Palumbo, F., Pecora, F., von Rump, S., Štimec, A., Ullberg, J., Ötslund, B.: GiraffPlus: a system for monitoring activities and physiological parameters and promoting social interaction for elderly. In: Hippe, Z.S., Kulikowski, J.L., Mroczek, T., Wtorek, J. (eds.) Human-Computer Systems Interaction: Backgrounds and Applications, vol. 3, pp. 261–271. Springer, New York (2014)
181. Lemlouma, T., Laborie, S., Roose, P.: Toward a context-aware and automatic evaluation of elderly dependency in smart homes and cities. In: World of Wireless, Mobile and Multimedia Networks (WoWMoM), 2013 IEEE 14th International Symposium and Workshops on a, pp. 1–6 (2013)
182. Broekens, J., Heerink, M., Rosendal, H.: Assistive social robots in elderly care: a review. Gerontechnology **8**(2), 94–103 (2009)
183. Tomita, M., Russ, L.S., Sridhar, R., Naughton M, B.J.: Smart home with healthcare technologies for community-dwelling older adults. In: Al-Qutayri, M.A. (ed.) Smart Home Systems. InTech. Rijeka (2010)
184. Bemelmans, R., Gelderblom, G.J., Jonker, P., Witte, L.: The potential of socially assistive robotics in care for elderly, a systematic review. In: Lamers, M.H., Verbeek, F.J. (eds.) Human-Robot Personal Relationships, vol. 59, pp. 83–89. Springer, Berlin/Heidelberg (2011)
185. Chang, W.-L., Sabanovic, S., Huber, L.: Use of seal-like robot PARO in sensory group therapy for older adults with dementia. In: 2013 8th ACM/IEEE International Conference on Human-Robot Interaction (HRI), pp. 101–102 (2013)
186. Nicolo, F., Parupati, S., Kulathumani, V., Schmid, N.A.: Near real-time face detection and recognition using a wireless camera network. Proc. SPIE **8392**, 1–10 (2012)
187. Watson, S., Wenzel, R.R., di Matteo, C., Meier, B., Lüscher, T.F.: Accuracy of a new wrist cuff oscillometric blood pressure device comparisons with intraarterial and mercury manometer measurements. Am. J. Hypertens. **11**(12), 1469–1474 (1998)
188. Yarows, S.A.: Comparison of the omron HEM-637 wrist monitor to the auscultation method with the wrist position sensor on or disabled*. Am. J. Hypertens. **17**(1), 54–58 (2004)
189. Uen, S., Weisser, B., Wieneke, P., Vetter, H., Mengden, T.: Evaluation of the performance of a wrist blood pressure measuring device with a position sensor compared to ambulatory 24-hour blood pressure measurements. Am. J. Hypertens. **15**(9), 787–792 (2002)
190. Uen, S., Weisser, B., Vetter, H., Mengden, T.: P-25: clinical evaluation of a wrist blood pressure device with an active positioning system by comparison with 24-H ambulatory blood pressure measurement. Am. J. Hypertens. **14**(S1), 37A–37A (2001)
191. Stergiou, G.S., Christodoulakis, G.R., Nasothimiou, E.G., Giovas, P.P., Kalogeropoulos, P.G.: Can validated wrist devices with position sensors replace arm devices for self-home blood pressure monitoring? A randomized crossover trial using ambulatory monitoring as reference. Am. J. Hypertens. **21**(7), 753–758 (2008)
192. Alahmadi A., Soh, B.: A smart approach towards a mobile e-health monitoring system architecture. In: 2011 International Conference on Research and Innovation in Information Systems (ICRIIS), pp. 1–5 (2011)
193. Tamura, T.: Home geriatric physiological measurements. Physiol. Meas. **33**(10), R47–R65 (2012)
194. Wang, S., Ji, L., Li, A., Wu, J.: Body sensor networks for ubiquitous healthcare. J. Control Theory Appl. **9**(1), 3–9 (2011)
195. Lin, Y.: A natural contact sensor paradigm for nonintrusive and real-time sensing of biosignals in human-machine interactions. IEEE Sens. J. **11**(3), 522–529 (2011)
196. Jacobsen, R.H., Kortermand, K., Zhang, Q., Toftegaard, T.S.: Understanding link behavior of non-intrusive wireless body sensor networks. Wirel. Pers. Commun. **64**(3), 561–582 (2012)
197. Baek, H.J., Chung, G.S., Kim, K.K., Park, K.S.: A smart health monitoring chair for nonintrusive measurement of biological signals. IEEE Trans. Inf. Technol. Biomed. **16**(1), 150–158 (2012)

198. Sullivan, A.M., Xia, H., McBride, J.C., Zhao, X.: Reconstruction of missing physiological signals using artificial neural networks. Comput. Cardiol. **37**, 317–320 (2010)
199. Dinesen, B., Sørensen, N., Østergaard, C.U.: Effect evaluation of the intelligent bed in a nursing home: the case of Tangshave nursing home. Department of Health Science and Technology, Aalborg University, Aalborg (2012)
200. Costa, Â., Castillo, J.C., Novais, P., Fernández-Caballero, A., Simoes, R.: Sensor-driven agenda for intelligent home care of the elderly. Expert Syst. Appl. **39**(15), 12192–12204 (2012)
201. Monekosso, D.N., Remagnino, P.: Monitoring behavior with an array of sensors. Comput. Intell. **23**(4), 420–438 (2007)
202. Helal, A., Cook, D.J., Schmalz, M.: Smart home-based health platform for behavioral monitoring and alteration of diabetes patients. J. Diabetes Sci. Technol. Online **3**(1), 141–148 (2009)
203. Jafari, R., Li, W., Bajcsy, R., Glaser, S., Sastry, S.: Physical activity monitoring for assisted living at home. In: Leonhardt, S., Falck, T., Mähönen, P. (eds.) 4th International Workshop on Wearable and Implantable Body Sensor Networks (BSN 2007), vol. 13, pp. 213–219. Springer, Berlin/Heidelberg (2007)
204. Kulkarni, P., Ozturk, Y.: mPHASiS: mobile patient healthcare and sensor information system. J. Netw. Comput. Appl. **34**(1), 402–417 (2011)
205. Williams, M.E., Owens, J.E., Parker, B.E., Granata, K.P.: A new approach to assessing function in elderly people. Trans. Am. Clin. Climatol. Assoc. **114**, 203–217 (2003)
206. Karunanithi, M.: Monitoring technology for the elderly patient. Expert Rev. Med. Devices **4**(2), 267–277 (2007)
207. Sanchez-Garcia, S., Garcia-Pena, C., Duque-Lopez, M.X., Juarez-Cedillo, T., Cortes-Nunez, A.R., Reyes-Beaman, S.: Anthropometric measures and nutritional status in a healthy elderly population. BMC Public Health **7**, 2 (2007)
208. Helal, S., Mann, W., El-Zabadani, H., King, J., Kaddoura, Y., Jansen, E.: The gator tech smart house: a programmable pervasive space. Computer **38**(3), 50–60 (2005)
209. Karottki, D.G., Spilak, M., Frederiksen, M., Gunnarsen, L., Brauner, E.V., Kolarik, B., Andersen, Z.J., Sigsgaard, T., Barregard, L., Strandberg, B., Sallsten, G., Møller, P., Loft, S.: An indoor air filtration study in homes of elderly: cardiovascular and respiratory effects of exposure to particulate matter. Environ. Health **12**(1), 116 (2013)
210. Dodd, E., Hawting, P., Horton, E., Karunanithi, M., Livingstone, A.: Australian community care experience on the design, development, deployment and evaluation of implementing the smarter safer homes platform. In: Geissbühler, A., Demongeot, J., Mokhtari, M., Abdulrazak, B., Aloulou, H. (eds.) Inclusive Smart Cities and e-Health, pp. 282–286. Springer International Publishing, Cham (2015)
211. McMichael, A.J., Woodruff, R.E., Hales, S.: Climate change and human health: present and future risks. Lancet **367**(9513), 859–869 (2006), 11
212. Sehili, M.A., Lecouteux, B., Vacher, M., Portet, F., Istrate, D., Dorizzi, B., Boudy, J.: Sound environment analysis in smart home. In: Paternò, F., de Ruyter, B., Markopoulos, P., Santoro, C., van Loenen, E., Luyten, K. (eds.) Ambient Intelligence, pp. 208–223. Springer, Berlin/Heidelberg (2012)
213. Corchado, J.M., Bajo, J., Tapia, D.I., Abraham, A.: Using heterogeneous wireless sensor networks in a telemonitoring system for healthcare. IEEE Trans. Inf. Technol. Biomed. **14**(2), 234–240 (2010)
214. Hensel, B.K., Demiris, G., Courtney, K.L.: Defining obtrusiveness in home telehealth technologies a conceptual framework. J. Am. Med. Inform. Assoc. **13**(4), 428–431 (2006)
215. Rahimi, S., Chan, A.D.C., Goubran, R.A.: Nonintrusive load monitoring of electrical devices in health smart homes. In: Instrumentation and Measurement Technology Conference (I2MTC), 2012 IEEE International, pp. 2313–2316 (2012)
216. Soltan, M., Pedram, M.: Durability of wireless networks of battery-powered devices. In: Proceedings of the 6th IEEE Conference on Consumer Communications and Networking Conference, pp. 263–268. Piscataway (2009)

217. Pensas, H., Raula, H., Vanhala, J.: Energy efficient sensor network with service discovery for smart home environments. In: Third International Conference on Sensor Technologies and Applications, 2009. SENSORCOMM '09, pp. 399–404 (2009)
218. Becker, E., Guerra-Filho, G., Makedon, F.: Automatic sensor placement in a 3D volume. In: Proceedings of the 2nd International Conference on Pervasive Technologies Related to Assistive Environments, vol. 8, pp. 36:1–36. New York (2009)
219. Banos, O., Toth, M.A., Damas, M., Pomares, H., Rojas, I.: Dealing with the effects of sensor displacement in wearable activity recognition. Sensors **14**(6), 9995–10023 (2014)
220. Uslu, G., Altun, O., Baydere, S.: A Bayesian approach for indoor human activity monitoring. In: 2011 11th International Conference on Hybrid Intelligent Systems (HIS), pp. 324–327 (2011)
221. Zhang, Y.: Real-time development of patient-specific alarm algorithms for critical care. In: 29th Annual International Conference of the IEEE Engineering in Medicine and Biology Society, 2007. EMBS 2007, pp. 4351–4354 (2007)
222. Cook, D.J., Crandall, A.S., Thomas, B.L., Krishnan, N.C.: CASAS: a smart home in a box. Computer **46**(7), 62–69 (2013)
223. Watrous, R., Towell, G.: A patient-adaptive neural network ECG patient monitoring algorithm. Comput. Cardiol. 229–232 (1995)
224. Liszka-Hackzell, J.: Categorization of fetal heart rate patterns using neural networks. Comput. Cardiol. 97–100 (1994)
225. Abouei, V., Sharifian, H., Towhidkhah, F., Nafisi, V., Abouie, H.: Using neural network in order to predict hypotension of hemodialysis patients. In: 2011 19th Iranian Conference on Electrical Engineering (ICEE), pp. 1–4 (2011)
226. Dawadi, P., Cook, D., Parsey, C., Schmitter-Edgecombe, M., Schneider, M.: An approach to cognitive assessment in smart home. In: Proceedings of the 2011 Workshop on Data Mining for Medicine and Healthcare, pp. 56–59. New York (2011)
227. Atoui, H., Fayn, J., Rubel, P.: A neural network approach for patient-specific 12-lead ECG synthesis in patient monitoring environments. Comput. Cardiol. **31**, 161–164 (2004)
228. Yu, M., Rhuma, A., Naqvi, S.M., Wang, L., Chambers, J.: A posture recognition-based fall detection system for monitoring an elderly person in a smart home environment. IEEE Trans. Inf. Technol. Biomed. **16**(6), 1274–1286 (2012)
229. Novak, M., Binas, M., Jakab, F.: Unobtrusive anomaly detection in presence of elderly in a smart-home environment. In: ELEKTRO, 2012, pp. 341–344 (2012)
230. Nazerfard, E., Das, B., Holder, L.B., Cook, D.J.: Conditional random fields for activity recognition in smart environments. In: Proceedings of the 1st ACM International Health Informatics Symposium, pp. 282–286. New York (2010)
231. Fleury, A., Noury, N., Vacher, M., Glasson, H., Seri, J.F.: Sound and speech detection and classification in a Health Smart Home. In: Conference Proceedings Annual International Conference IEEE Engineering in Medical and Biology Society, vol. 2008, pp. 4644–4647 (2008)
232. Sánchez, M., Martín, P., Álvarez, L., Alonso, V., Zato, C., Pedrero, A., Bajo, J.: A new adaptive algorithm for detecting falls through mobile devices. In: Corchado, J.M., Pérez, J.B., Hallenborg, K., Golinska, P., Corchuelo, R. (eds.) Trends in Practical Applications of Agents and Multiagent Systems, pp. 17–24. Springer, Berlin/Heidelberg (2011)
233. Mahmoud, S.M., Lotfi, A., Langensiepen, C.: Behavioural pattern identification in a smart home using binary similarity and dissimilarity measures. In: 2011 7th International Conference on Intelligent Environments (IE), pp. 55–60 (2011)
234. Albert, M.V., Kording, K., Herrmann, M., Jayaraman, A.: Fall classification by machine learning using mobile phones. PLoS One **7**(5), e36556 (2012)
235. Snijders, A.H., van de Warrenburg, B.P., Giladi, N., Bloem, B.R.: Neurological gait disorders in elderly people: clinical approach and classification. Lancet Neurol. **6**(1), 63–74 (2007)
236. Roark, B., Mitchell, M., Hosom, J., Hollingshead, K., Kaye, J.: Spoken language derived measures for detecting mild cognitive impairment. IEEE Trans. Audio Speech Lang. Process. **19**(7), 2081–2090 (2011)

237. Khawandi, S., Ballit, A., Daya, B.: Applying machine learning algorithm in fall detection monitoring system. In: 2013 5th International Conference on Computational Intelligence and Communication Networks (CICN), pp. 247–250 (2013)
238. Oguz Kansiz, A., Amac Guvensan, M., Irem Turkmen, H.: Selection of time-domain features for fall detection based on supervised learning. In: Proceedings of the World Congress on Engineering and Computer Science 2013, vol. 2, pp. 796–801. San Francisco (2013)
239. Hong, H.G., He, X.: Prediction of functional status for the elderly based on a new ordinal regression model. J. Am. Stat. Assoc. **105**(491), 930–941 (2010)
240. Rose, S.: Mortality risk score prediction in an elderly population using machine learning. Am. J. Epidemiol. **177**(5), 443–452 (2013)
241. Cheng, F., Zhao, Z.: Machine learning-based prediction of drug–drug interactions by integrating drug phenotypic, therapeutic, chemical, and genomic properties. J. Am. Med. Inform. Assoc. **21**(e2), e278–e286 (2014)
242. Yang, Y., Hauptmann, A., Chen, M., Cai, Y., Bharucha, A., Wactlar, H.: Learning to predict health status of geriatric patients from observational data. In: 2012 IEEE Symposium on Computational Intelligence in Bioinformatics and Computational Biology (CIBCB), pp. 127–134 (2012)
243. Marschollek, M., Rehwald, A., Wolf, K.-H., Gietzelt, M., Nemitz, G., zu Schwabedissen, H.M., Schulze, M.: Sensors vs. experts – a performance comparison of sensor-based fall risk assessment vs. conventional assessment in a sample of geriatric patients. BMC Med. Inform. Decis. Mak. **11**(1), 1–7 (2011)
244. Marschollek, M., Gövercin, M., Rust, S., Gietzelt, M., Schulze, M., Wolf, K.-H., Steinhagen-Thiessen, E.: Mining geriatric assessment data for in-patient fall prediction models and high-risk subgroups. BMC Med. Inform. Decis. Mak. **12**(1), 1–6 (2012)
245. Shankle, W.R., Romney, A.K., Hara, J., Fortier, D., Dick, M.B., Chen, J.M., Chan, T., Sun, X.: Methods to improve the detection of mild cognitive impairment. Proc. Natl. Acad. Sci. U. S. A. **102**(13), 4919–4924 (2005)
246. Kalra, L., Zhao, X., Soto, A.J., Milios, E.: Detection of daily living activities using a two-stage Markov model. J. Ambient Intell. Smart Environ. **5**(3), 273–285 (2013)
247. van Kasteren, T., Noulas, A., Englebienne, G., Kröse, B.: Accurate activity recognition in a home setting. In: Proceedings of the 10th International Conference on Ubiquitous Computing, pp. 1–9 (2008)
248. Reiss, A., Stricker, D.: Creating and benchmarking a new dataset for physical activity monitoring. In: Proceedings of the 5th International Conference on Pervasive Technologies Related to Assistive Environments, pp. 40:1–40:8 (2012)
249. Li, L.-N., Ouyang, J.-H., Chen, H.-L., Liu, D.-Y.: A computer aided diagnosis system for thyroid disease using extreme learning machine. J. Med. Syst. **36**(5), 3327–3337 (2012)
250. Petersen, J., Larimer, N., Kaye, J.A., Pavel, M., Hayes, T.L.: SVM to detect the presence of visitors in a smart home environment. In: 2012 Annual International Conference of the IEEE Engineering in Medicine and Biology Society (EMBC), pp. 5850–5853 (2012)
251. John D. Lafferty, Andrew McCallum, Fernando C. N. Pereira. Conditional random fields: Probabilistic models for segmenting and labeling sequence data. In Carla E. Brodley, Andrea Pohoreckyj Danyluk (eds.) Proceedings of the Eighteenth International Conference on Machine Learning (ICML '01), Morgan Kaufmann Publishers Inc., San Francisco, pp. 282–289, (2001)
252. Vinh, L.T., Lee, S., Le, H.X., Ngo, H.Q., Kim, H.I., Han, M., Lee, Y.-K.: Semi-Markov conditional random fields for accelerometer-based activity recognition. Appl. Intell. **35**(2), 226–241 (2011)
253. Šmuc, T., Gamberger, D., Krstačić, G.: Combining unsupervised and supervised machine learning in analysis of the CHD patient database. In: Quaglini, S., Barahona, P., Andreassen, S. (eds.) Artificial Intelligence in Medicine, pp. 109–112. Springer, Berlin/Heidelberg (2001)
254. Obayya, M., Abou-Chadi, F.: Data fusion for heart diseases classification using multi-layer feed forward neural network. In: International Conference on Computer Engineering Systems, 2008. ICCES 2008, pp. 67–70 (2008)

255. Obo, T., Kubota, N.: Remote monitoring and control using smart phones and sensor networks. In: 2012 IEEE 1st Global Conference on Consumer Electronics (GCCE), pp. 466–469 (2012)
256. Ravi, N., Dandekar, N., Mysore, P., Littman, M.L.: Activity recognition from accelerometer data. In: Proceedings of the Seventeenth Conference on Innovative Applications of Artificial Intelligence (IAAI), pp. 1541–1546 (2005)
257. Bao, L., Intille, S.S.: Activity Recognition from User-Annotated Acceleration Data, pp. 1–17. Springer, Berlin Heidelberg (2004)
258. Cherkassky, M.: Application of machine learning methods to medical diagnosis. Chance **22**(1), 42–50 (2009)
259. Clifton, L., Clifton, D.A., Pimentel, M., Watkinson, P.J., Tarassenko, L.: Gaussian processes for personalized e-Health monitoring with wearable sensors. IEEE Trans. Biomed. Eng. **60**(1), 193–197 (2013)
260. Wong, D., Clifton, D.A., Tarassenko, L.: Probabilistic detection of vital sign abnormality with Gaussian process regression In: 2012 IEEE 12th International Conference on Bioinformatics Bioengineering (BIBE), pp. 187–192 (2012)
261. Chen, J., Zhang, J., Kam, A.H., Shue, L.: An automatic acoustic bathroom monitoring system. IEEE Int. Symp. Circuits Syst. **2**, 1750–1753 (2005)
262. Rasmussen, C.E., Williams, C.K.I.: Gaussian Processes for Machine Learning. MIT Press, Cambridge, MA (2006)
263. Laydrus, N.C., Ambikairajah, E., Celler, B.: Automated sound analysis system for home telemonitoring using shifted delta cepstral features. In: 2007 15th International Conference on Digital Signal Processing, pp. 135–138 (2007)
264. Libal, V., Ramabhadran, B., Mana, N., Pianesi, F., Chippendale, P., Lanz, O., Potamianos, G.: Multimodal classification of activities of daily living inside smart homes. In: Omatu, S., Rocha, M.P., Bravo, J., Fernández, F., Corchado, E., Bustillo, A., Corchado, J.M. (eds.) Distributed Computing, Artificial Intelligence, Bioinformatics, Soft Computing, and Ambient Assisted Living, pp. 687–694. Springer, Berlin/Heidelberg (2009)
265. Zhuang, X., Huang, J., Potamianos, G., Hasegawa-Johnson, M.: Acoustic fall detection using Gaussian mixture models and GMM supervectors. In: IEEE International Conference on Acoustics, Speech and Signal Processing, 2009. ICASSP 2009, pp. 69–72 (2009)
266. Salama, M.A., Hassanien, A.E., Fahmy, A.A.: Deep belief network for clustering and classification of a continuous data. In: 2010 IEEE International Symposium on Signal Processing and Information Technology (ISSPIT), pp. 473–477 (2010)
267. Shi, J.Q., Murray-Smith, R., Titterington, D.M.: Hierarchical Gaussian process mixtures for regression. Stat. Comput. **15**(1), 31–41 (2005)
268. McKenna, S.J., Charif, H.N.: Summarising contextual activity and detecting unusual inactivity in a supportive home environment. Pattern Anal. Appl. **7**(4), 386–401 (2004)
269. Wang, L., Gu, T., Tao, X., Chen, H., Lu, J.: Multi-user activity recognition in a smart home. In: Chen, L., Nugent, C.D., Biswas, J., Hoey, J. (eds.) Activity Recognition in Pervasive Intelligent Environments, pp. 59–81. Atlantis Press, Paris (2011)
270. Tong, Y., Chen, R.: Latent-dynamic conditional random fields for recognizing activities in smart homes. J. Ambient Intell. Smart Environ. **6**(1), 39–55 (2014)
271. Bishop, C.M.: Pattern Recognition and Machine Learning, 1st edn. 2006. Corr. 2nd printing 2011. Springer, New York (2007)
272. Kononenko, I.: Machine learning for medical diagnosis: history, state of the art and perspective. Artif. Intell. Med. **23**(1), 89–109 (2001)
273. Settles, B.: From theories to queries: active learning in practice. Act. Learn. Exp. Des. W. **16**, 1–18 (2011)
274. López, V., Fernández, A., Moreno-Torres, J.G., Herrera, F.: Analysis of preprocessing vs. cost-sensitive learning for imbalanced classification. Open problems on intrinsic data characteristics. Expert Syst. Appl. **39**(7), 6585–6608 (2012)

275. Das, B., Krishnan, N.C., Cook, D.J.: Handling class overlap and imbalance to detect prompt situations in smart homes. In: 2013 IEEE 13th International Conference on Data Mining Workshops (ICDMW), pp. 266–273 (2013)
276. Chawla, N.V., Bowyer, K.W., Hall, L.O., Kegelmeyer, W.P.: SMOTE: synthetic minority over-sampling technique. J. Artif. Intell. Res. **16**, 321–357 (2002)
277. Zeng, Z., Ji, Q.: Knowledge based activity recognition with dynamic Bayesian network. In: Daniilidis, K., Maragos, P., Paragios, N. (eds.) Computer Vision – ECCV 2010, pp. 532–546. Springer, Berlin/Heidelberg (2010)
278. Ozcift, A., Gulten, A.: Classifier ensemble construction with rotation forest to improve medical diagnosis performance of machine learning algorithms. Comput. Methods Programs Biomed. **104**(3), 443–451 (2011)
279. Meyfroidt, G., Güiza, F., Ramon, J., Bruynooghe, M.: Machine learning techniques to examine large patient databases. Best Pract. Res. Clin. Anaesthesiol. **23**(1), 127–143 (2009)
280. WHO: WHO | Medical Device – Full Definition. http://www.who.int/medical_devices/full_deffinition/en/. Accessed 10 Sept 2015
281. C. for D. and R. Health: FDA basics – are medical devices regulated for non-medical reasons? http://www.fda.gov/AboutFDA/Transparency/Basics/ucm302659.htm. Accessed 10 Sept 2015
282. Council of the European Communities: Council Directive 93/42/EEC concerning medical devices. Off. J. 1–60 (2007)
283. European Commission: Implementation of Directive 2007/47/EC amending Directives 90/385/EEC, 93/42/EEC and 98/8/EC. European Commission (2009)
284. MDC Medical Device Certification Gmbh: Basic Information about the European Directive 93/42/EEC on Medical Devices. 13 Nov 2009
285. International Organization for Standardization: ISO 13485:2003 – medical devices – quality management systems – requirements for regulatory purposes. http://www.iso.org/iso/home/store/catalogue_tc/catalogue_detail.htm?csnumber=36786 (2003). Accessed 11 Sept 2015
286. International Organization for Standardization: ISO 14971:2007 – medical devices – application of risk management to medical devices. http://www.iso.org/iso/catalogue_detail?csnumber=38193 (2007). Accessed 11 Sept 2015.
287. International Electrotechnical Commission: IEC 60601–1:2015 SER Series | Medical electrical equipment – ALL PARTS. https://webstore.iec.ch/publication/2612 (2015). Accessed 11 Sept 2015
288. International Electrotechnical Commission: IECEE TRF 60601-1-2:2015 | Medical electrical equipment – Part 1–2: general requirements for basic safety and essential performance – collateral standard: electromagnetic disturbances – requirements and tests. https://webstore.iec.ch/publication/8218 (2015). Accessed 17 Sept 2015
289. International Electrotechnical Commission: IECEE TRF 60601-1-6:2014 | Medical electrical equipment – Part 1–6: general requirements for basic safety and essential performance – collateral standard: usability. https://webstore.iec.ch/publication/8225 (2014). Accessed 17 Sept 2015
290. IEC 60601-1-8:2006 – Medical electrical equipment – Part 1–8: general requirements for basic safety and essential performance – collateral standard: general requirements, tests and guidance for alarm systems in medical electrical equipment and medical electrical systems. http://www.iso.org/iso/home/store/catalogue_tc/catalogue_detail.htm?csnumber=41986 (2006). Accessed 11 Sept 2015
291. International Electrotechnical Commission: IEC 60601-1-9:2007 | Medical electrical equipment – Part 1–9: general requirements for basic safety and essential performance – collateral standard: requirements for environmentally conscious design. https://webstore.iec.ch/publication/2601 (2007). Accessed 17 Sept 2015
292. International Electrotechnical Commission: IEC 60601-1-11:2015 – medical electrical equipment – Part 1–11: general requirements for basic safety and essential performance – collateral standard: requirements for medical electrical equipment and medical electrical systems used in the home healthcare environment. http://www.iso.org/iso/home/store/catalogue_tc/catalogue_detail.htm?csnumber=65529 (2015). Accessed 11 Sept 2015

293. International Electrotechnical Commission: IEC 62304:2006 – medical device software – software life cycle processes. http://www.iso.org/iso/catalogue_detail.htm?csnumber=38421 (2006). Accessed 16 Sept 2015
294. International Organization for Standardization: ISO 10993–1:2009 – biological evaluation of medical devices – Part 1: evaluation and testing within a risk management process. http://www.iso.org/iso/catalogue_detail.htm?csnumber=44908 (2009). Accessed 17 Sept 2015
295. International Organization for Standardization: ISO 15223–1:2012 – medical devices – symbols to be used with medical device labels, labelling and information to be supplied – Part 1: general requirements. http://www.iso.org/iso/catalogue_detail.htm?csnumber=50335 (2012). Accessed 17 Sept 2015
296. British Standards Institution: BS EN 1041:2008+A1:2013. http://www.techstreet.com/products/1867028#jumps (2013). Accessed 17 Sept 2015
297. International Organization for Standardization: ISO 14155:2011 – clinical investigation of medical devices for human subjects – good clinical practice. http://www.iso.org/iso/catalogue_detail?csnumber=45557 (2011). Accessed 17 Sept 2015
298. European Commission: MEDDEV 2.7.1 Rev.3:2009 guidelines on medical devices. Clinical evaluation: a guide for manufacturers and notified bodies. GHTF (2009)
299. International Electrotechnical Commission: IEC 62366–1:2015 – medical devices – part 1: application of usability engineering to medical devices. http://www.iso.org/iso/catalogue_detail.htm?csnumber=63179 (2015). Accessed 11 Sept 2015
300. International Organization for Standardization: ISO 27001 – information security management. http://www.iso.org/iso/home/standards/management-standards/iso27001.htm (2013). Accessed 16 Sept 2015
301. International Organization for Standardization: ISO/IEC 25010:2011 – systems and software engineering – systems and software quality requirements and evaluation (SQuaRE) – system and software quality models. http://www.iso.org/iso/home/store/catalogue_ics/catalogue_detail_ics.htm?csnumber=35733 (2011). Accessed 16 Sept 2015
302. Medical Devices – European Commission. http://ec.europa.eu/growth/single-market/european-standards/harmonised-standards/medical-devices/index_en.htm (2015). Accessed 11 Sept 2015
303. Yogesan, K., Brett, P., Gibbons, M.C.: Handbook of Digital Homecare. Springer Science & Business Media, Berlin (2009)

Chapter 5
Datasets

Abstract Publicly available datasets constitute the ground to evaluate and compare the performance of proposed approaches for monitoring older patients at home. In this chapter, we shed light on the importance of using datasets as a benchmarking tool for comparing various monitoring techniques for detecting the health threats, which we discussed in the previous chapters. The methods, which are tested by using a standard publicly available dataset as a benchmark, are considered to be more reliable and are more likely to be accepted by the scientific community for their claimed results. Therefore, we summarize the references of available datasets, which are relevant to the field of automatic monitoring of older patients.

Keywords Patient monitoring dataset • Activity recognition dataset • Fall detection dataset • Wandering detection dataset • Audiovisual data • Benchmarking

In the context of audiovisual content-based monitoring, a dataset contain audio and video clips of human body parts and/or activities in experimental or real-life environments. In the context of measuring movements and locations of patients, for example, by means of radio-frequency sensors, infrared detectors, or inertial sensors, a dataset usually contains annotated recordings of a finite set of specific ADLs. Sampling rate of these recordings may vary, depending on the monitoring equipment, and numeric timestamps are usually assigned to every instance of the recorded data. The attributes of those datasets can be very different and may simultaneously contain both numeric and categorical variables. Every dataset should in principle contain detailed description about how the data was collected and annotated. Often the data is already preprocessed. Therefore, the detailed description of those preprocessing steps should be included in the dataset description as well, often accompanied with available program source code. Most important dataset descriptions usually are included in a so-called “readme” file.

Though a vast body of literature has been produced for older patient monitoring, in fact, a few methods are tested on real older patients’ data. Most of the methods used their own configuration of sensors for data acquisition and young people as actors in a laboratory environment to create scenes and tested the system by their custom dataset. The datasets are not only varying in number and placement of sensors but

J. Klonovs et al., *Distributed Computing and Monitoring Technologies for Older Patients*, SpringerBriefs in Computer Science,
DOI 10.1007/978-3-319-27024-1_5

also varying by objective of data collection (e.g., fall detection or specific set of ADLs detection), environmental description, and subjects' behavior. Thus, the results from one method tested on a custom dataset are not comparable with the results of another method tested on some other custom datasets. Also, the results from a method that is tested on the data collected from young volunteers may significantly differ for older adults, because of dissimilarity between the data obtained from real seniors and the data obtained from young volunteers in the laboratory. For example, a real fall of an older adult and an acted fall of a young man in the laboratory may not "look" similar [1]. Thus, it is very difficult to predict the performance of a proposed method in a real-life scenario. Additionally, making a dataset publicly available might be very difficult due to the privacy policies of personal data [2]. Thus, only few publicly available datasets can be obtained from the literature. In previous reviews, Aggarwal et al. [3] divided the available datasets for human activity monitoring in three broad themes: action recognition datasets, surveillance datasets, and movie datasets. However, only the action recognition datasets are well suited for in-home activity monitoring. On the other hand, Popoola et al. [4] listed a number of publicly available datasets from in-home scenarios for fall detection, kitchen activities, audiovisual activities, and daily activities. A summary of well-known, publicly available and generic action recognition dataset (not specifically for geriatric patients) is presented in [5]. None of these reviews focused on datasets that are strictly relevant to geriatric patient monitoring. Thus, this chapter provides a description of important datasets used in the literature. Though some datasets are collected by using multimodal sensors and included the scenarios of human activity recognition, e.g., acoustic event detection datasets in [5–8] and visual activity detection dataset in [9], we do not include summaries of these datasets in our book, because of the too broad activity classes considered in these datasets and they are not relevant to geriatric patient monitoring.

It is also worth noting that the first study, which proposed to use datasets as a benchmarking tool, was [10]; however in their rich dataset, which focused mainly on activity recognition, they did not include data on vital signs that are prerequisites for assessing the health state of patients and thus are very important for finding correlation between ADL data and vital sign data (e.g., which can be used to validate ADL data).

Table 5.1 lists the datasets and their key characteristics. We mention the datasets either by the names given by the creators of the datasets or by the first author of the articles that introduced the dataset. The description of the datasets includes the overall data acquisition environment, dataset size, and types of dataset (annotated/non-annotated or real-life/laboratory implementation). Column 4 states the intended application of the dataset collection, e.g., activity recognition, fall detection, wandering detection, and elopement detection. Column 5 mentions the subjects used in the scene to create these datasets. Column 6 indicates the types of sensors used in each dataset collection. The last column in Table 5.1 states whether the dataset is available online or not. We write "Yes" for the datasets which are already available online or can be acquired by filling up an online requisition form. From Table 5.1, it is observed that some datasets, such as "Multi-view fall dataset," were used in a number of works. We found only one dataset in [24] that considered the issue of

Table 5.1 The available datasets relevant to the field of automatic monitoring of older patients

No.	Dataset name/first author	Description	Objective(s)	Subjects	Sensors	Online
1	PLIA1 and PLIA2 [11]	Two annotated datasets of ADLs of several hours	Activity recognition/unusual activity detection	Young actors	Multi-sensors including microphone and video cameras	Yes
2	Tap30F and Tap80F [12]	An annotated dataset of 14 days with activities of two subjects in private homes	Activity recognition/health threatening conditions detection	A 30 years and a 80 years old women	Environmental stage change sensors	No
3	WSU CASAS [13]	Activities performed by two residents over three months in a test bed smart apartment	Activity recognition/unusual activity detection	Two young actors	Environmental stage change sensors	Yes
4	A. Reiss [14]	A dataset containing both indoor and outdoor activities, where indoor activities are relevant to our topic	Activity recognition	Nine young actors	Wearable sensors	Yes
5	TK26M and TK57M [15]	An annotated dataset of activities of two subjects in a private apartment and a house	Activity recognition/health threatening conditions detection	A 26 years and a 57 years old men	Environmental stage change sensors	Yes
6	Multi-view fall dataset [16–22]	24 fall incidences in 24 scenarios and includes different kinds of fall, e.g., forward and backward fall	Fall detection	Young actors	Video cameras	Yes

(continued)

Table 5.1 (continued)

No.	Dataset name/first author	Description	Objective(s)	Subjects	Sensors	Online
7	T. Liu [23]	12 h of video data containing seven previously instructed activities and fall events	Activity recognition/unusual activity detection/Fall detection	Young actors	Video camera	Yes
8	Nursing Home Dataset [24]	13,800 camera hours of video (25 days x 24 h per day x 23 cameras) obtained from a test bed developed in a dementia unit of a real nursing home	Elopement (leaving home) detection/Unusual activity detection/ Wandering detection	15 elderly dementia patients	Video camera	No
9	C. Zhang [25]	A dataset of 200 video sequences with RGB-D information in three conditions: subject is within 4 m with/without enough illumination and subject is out of 4 m distance from the camera	Fall detection	Young actors	RGB-D camera	No
10	D. Anderson [26]	18 video sequences that are captured in 3 fps capture rate and a total of 5512 frames (30 min)	Fall detection	Two young actors	Video camera	No

11	I. Charfi [27]	An annotated dataset of 191 videos that are collected by varying different environmental attributes	Fall detection	Young actors	Video camera	Yes
12	CompanionAble [28, 29]	An annotated dataset containing audio files of different environmental and life sound classes	Sound event detection for remote monitoring	Young actors	Microphone	Yes
13	B. Bonroy [30]	An annotated dataset of 15 min video recording containing 80 different events captured by two cameras	Detection of discomfort in demented elderly	Six demented older patients	Video cameras	No
14	SAR [31]	A non-annotated video dataset that is collected from real elderly living at home	Activity recognition/unusual activity detection	Six older adults (age >65 years and ten days video data for each person)	Video cameras	Yes
15	E. Syngelakis [32]	An annotated dataset of 200 video clips containing both fall and non-fall events in different variations of laboratory environment	Fall detection	Three young actors	Video camera	No

(continued)

Table 5.1 (continued)

No.	Dataset name/first author	Description	Objective(s)	Subjects	Sensors	Online
16	R. Romdhane [33]	A video dataset of real elderly which are captured by two cameras while performing ADLs in a nursing home	Activity recognition/unusual activity detection	Three elderly having Alzheimer's disease (Two male and one female)	Video cameras	No
17	C. F. C. Junior [34]	A dataset of ADLs acquired by multiple sensors in a nursing home	Activity recognition/unusual activity detection	Four healthy and Five elderly people with MCI (Mild Cognitive Impairment)	Multiple sensor including video cameras	No
18	GER'HOME dataset [35, 36]	A dataset of ADLs acquired by multiple sensors in an experimental apartment	Activity recognition/Unusual activity detection	14 elderly people (aged from 60 to 85 years), each one during 4 h	Multiple sensor including four video cameras and a number of environmental stage change sensors	Yes
19	REALDISP dataset [37, 38]	A dataset of 33 different physical activities acquired in three different scenarios by nine inertial sensors for investigating the effects of sensor displacement in the activity recognition process in real-world settings	Determining optimal sensor positioning for activity recognition and benchmarking activity recognition algorithms	17 young healthy actors (age ranging from 22 to 37 years old)	Multiple wearable sensors on nine different body parts: 3D accelerometers, 3D gyroscopes, 3D magnetic field orientation sensors, 4D quarterions	Yes

20	B. Kaluža et al. [39]	A localization dataset for posture reconstruction and person activity recognition, including falling	Activity recognition and fall detection	Five young healthy actors	Attached four radio-frequency body tags (chest, belt and two angles) recording 3D coordinates	Yes
21	D. Cook et al. [40]	A dataset with IADLs and memory in older adulthood and dementia patients in a real-home setting	Mild cognitive impairment (MCI) and dementia detection using IADL data, such as cooking and using the telephone	400 subjects, including healthy younger adults and older adults with MCI and dementia	Multimodal sensors: motion detectors, door sensors, stove sensors, temperature sensors, water sensors, etc.	Yes

elopement and wandering detection. Unfortunately, most of the datasets are developed by employing young actors instead of older adults or geriatric patients. Only few datasets are developed by employing older patients. In addition to Table 5.1, other relevant collections of public datasets are available online [41, 42].

References

1. Dalton, J., McGrath, M., Pavel, M., Jimison, H.: Home and mobile monitoring systems. CAPSIL, School of Public Health, Physiotherapy, and Population Science, Dublin, Ireland, Deliverable, Roadmap Draft 3.12, May 2009
2. Bharucha, A.J., London, A.J., Barnard, D., Wactlar, H., Dew, M.A., Reynolds 3rd C.F.: Ethical considerations in the conduct of electronic surveillance research. J. Law Med. Ethics J. Am. Soc. Law Med. Ethics, 34(3), 611–619, 482, (2006)
3. Aggarwal, J.K., Ryoo, M.S.: Human activity analysis: a review. ACM Comput. Surv. **43**(3), 16:1–16:43 (2011)
4. Popoola, O.P., Wang, K.: Video-based abnormal human behavior recognition: a review. IEEE Trans. Syst. Man Cybern. Part C Appl. Rev. **42**(6), 865–878 (2012)
5. Ahad, M.A.R., Tan, J., Kim, H., Ishikawa, S.: Action dataset – a survey. In 2011 Proceedings of SICE Annual Conference (SICE), Tokyo, Japan, pp. 1650–1655 (2011)
6. Dikmen, O., Mesaros, A.: Sound event detection using non-negative dictionaries learned from annotated overlapping events. In: 2013 IEEE Workshop on Applications of Signal Processing to Audio and Acoustics (WASPAA), pp. 1–4 (2013)
7. Mesaros, A., Heittola, T., Eronen, A., Virtanen, T.: Acoustic event detection in real life recordings. In: 18th European Signal Processing Conference, pp. 1267–1271 (2010)
8. Vuegen, L., Broeck, B.V.D., Karsmakers, P., Hamme, H.V., Vanrumste, B.: Automatic monitoring of activities of daily living based on real-life acoustic sensor data: a~preliminary study. Proc. Fourth Workshop Speech Lang. Process. Assist. Technol. 113–118 (2013)
9. Ni, B., Wang, G., Moulin, P.: RGBD-HuDaAct: a color-depth video database for human daily activity recognition. In 2011 IEEE International Conference on Computer Vision Workshops (ICCV Workshops), pp. 1147–1153. Barcelona, ESP (2011)
10. Roggen, D., Calatroni, A., Rossi, M., Holleczek, T., F{ö}rster, K., Tr{ö}ster, G., Lukowicz, P., Bannach, D., Pirkl, G., Ferscha, A., Doppler, J., Holzmann, C., Kurz, M., Holl, G., Chavarriaga, R., Creatura, M., Del,: Collecting complex activity data sets in highly rich networked sensor environments. Presented at the Proceedings of the 7th International Conference on Networked Sensing Systems (INSS), Kassel, Germany (2010)
11. Intille, S.S., Larson, K., Tapia, E.M., Beaudin, J.S., Kaushik, P., Nawyn, J., Rockinson, R.: Using a live-in laboratory for ubiquitous computing research. In: Fishkin, K.P., Schiele, B., Nixon, P., Quigley, A. (eds.) Pervasive Computing, pp. 349–365. Springer, Berlin/Heidelberg (2006)
12. Tapia, E.M., Intille, S.S., Larson, K.: Activity recognition in the home using simple and ubiquitous sensors. In: Ferscha, A., Mattern, F. (eds.) Pervasive Computing, pp. 158–175. Springer, Berlin/Heidelberg (2004)
13. Kadouche, R., Pigot, H., Abdulrazak, B., Giroux, S.: User's behavior classification model for smart houses occupant prediction. In: Chen, L., Nugent, C.D., Biswas, J., Hoey, J. (eds.) Activity Recognition in Pervasive Intelligent Environments, pp. 149–164. Atlantis Press, Paris (2011)
14. Reiss, A., Stricker, D.: Creating and benchmarking a new dataset for physical activity monitoring. In: Proceedings of the 5th International Conference on PErvasive Technologies Related to Assistive Environments, pp. 40:1–40:8. Heraklion, GRC (2012)
15. van Kasteren, T.L.M., Englebienne, G., Kröse, B.J.A.: An activity monitoring system for elderly care using generative and discriminative models. Pers. Ubiquit Comput. **14**(6), 489–498 (2010)

16. Yogameena, B., Deepika, G., Mehjabeen, J.: RVM based human fall analysis for video surveillance applications. Res. J. Appl. Sci. Eng. Technol. **4**(24), 5361–5366 (2012)
17. Auvinet, E., Rougier, C., Meunier, J., St-Arnaud, A., Rousseau, J.: Multiple cameras fall dataset. DIRO-Univ. Montr. Tech Rep **1350** (2010)
18. Auvinet, E., Multon, F., Saint-Arnaud, A., Rousseau, J., Meunier, J.: Fall detection with multiple cameras: an occlusion-resistant method based on 3-d silhouette vertical distribution. Inf. Technol. Biomed. IEEE Trans. On **15**(2), 290–300 (2011)
19. Hung, D.H., Saito, H.: The estimation of heights and occupied areas of humans from two orthogonal views for fall detection. 電気学会論文誌 C 電子・情報・システム部門誌 **133**(1), 117–127 (2013)
20. Hung, D.H., Saito, H.: Fall detection with two cameras based on occupied area. In: Proceedings of 18th Japan-Korea Joint Workshop on Frontier in Computer Vision, pp. 33–39 (2012)
21. Rougier, C., St-Arnaud, A., Rousseau, J., Meunier, J.: Video surveillance for fall detection. INTECH Open Access Publisher (2011)
22. Rougier, C., Meunier, J., St-Arnaud, A., Rousseau, J.: Robust video surveillance for fall detection based on human shape deformation. IEEE Trans. Circuits Syst. Video Technol. **21**(5), 611–622 (2011)
23. Liu, T., Yao, H., Ji, R., Liu, Y., Liu, X., Sun, X., Xu, P., Zhang, Z.: Vision-based semi-supervised homecare with spatial constraint. In: Advances in Multimedia Information Processing-PCM 2008. pp. 416–425. Springer (2008)
24. Chen, M.-Y., Hauptmann, A., Bharucha, A., Wactlar, H., Yang, Y.: Human activity analysis for geriatric care in nursing homes. In: The Era of Interactive Media, pp. 53–61. Springer, New York (2013)
25. Zhang, C., Tian, Y., Capezuti, E.: Privacy preserving automatic fall detection for elderly using RGBD cameras. Springer, Berlin (2012)
26. Anderson, D., Luke, R., Skubic, M., Keller, J.M., Rantz, M., Aud, M.: Evaluation of a video based fall recognition system for elders using voxel space. Gerontechnology **7**(2), 68 (2008)
27. Charfi, I., Miteran, J., Dubois, J., Atri, M., Tourki, R.: Definition and performance evaluation of a robust SVM based fall detection solution. In 2012 Eighth International Conference on Signal Image Technology and Internet Based Systems (SITIS), pp. 218–224. Naples, Italy (2012)
28. Rougui, J.E., Istrate, D., Souidene, W.: Audio sound event identification for distress situations and context awareness In: Annual International Conference of the IEEE Engineering in Medicine and Biology Society, 2009. EMBC 2009. pp. 3501–3504. Minneapolis (2009)
29. Montalvao, J., Istrate, D., Boudy, J., Mouba, J.: Sound event detection in remote health care-small learning datasets and over constrained Gaussian mixture models. In Engineering in Medicine and Biology Society (EMBC), 2010 Annual International Conference of the IEEE, pp. 1146–1149. Buenos Aires, Argentina (2010)
30. Bonroy, B., Schiepers, P., Leysens, G., Miljkovic, D., Wils, M., De Maesschalck, L., Quanten, S., Triau, E., Exadaktylos, V., Berckmans, D., and others: Acquiring a dataset of labeled video images showing discomfort in demented elderly. Telemedicine E-Health 15(4), 370–378 (2009)
31. Cheng, H., Liu, Z., Zhao, Y., Ye, G., Sun, X.: Real world activity summary for senior home monitoring. Multimed. Tools Appl. **70**(1), 177–197 (2014)
32. Syngelakis, E., Collomosse, J.: A bag of features approach to ambient fall detection for domestic elder-care (2011)
33. Romdhane, R., Mulin, E., Derreumeaux, A., Zouba, N., Piano, J., Lee, L., Leroi, I., Mallea, P., David, R., Thonnat, M., et al. Automatic video monitoring system for assessment of Alzheimer's disease symptoms. J. Nutr. Health Aging 16(3), 213–218 (2012)
34. Crispim-Junior, C.F., Bremond, F., Joumier, V.: A multi-sensor approach for activity recognition in older patients. Presented at the Second International Conference on Ambient Computing, Applications, Services and Technologies – AMBIENT 2012 (2012)
35. Zouba, N., Bremond, F., Thonnat, M.: An activity monitoring system for real elderly at home: validation study. In: 2010 Seventh IEEE International Conference on Advanced Video and Signal Based Surveillance (AVSS), pp. 278–285 (2010)
36. Valentin, N.Z.E.: Multisensor fusion for monitoring elderly activities at home. Université Nice Sophia Antipolis (2010)

37. Baños, O., Damas, M., Pomares, H., Rojas, I., Tóth, M.A., Amft, O.: A benchmark dataset to evaluate sensor displacement in activity recognition. In: Proceedings of the 2012 ACM Conference on Ubiquitous Computing, New York, pp. 1026–1035 (2012)
38. Banos, O., Toth, M.A., Damas, M., Pomares, H., Rojas, I.: Dealing with the effects of sensor displacement in wearable activity recognition. Sensors **14**(6), 9995–10023 (2014)
39. Kaluža, B., Cvetković, B., Dovgan, E., Gjoreski, H., Gams, M., Luštrek, M., Mirchevska, V.: A multi-agent care system to support independent living. Int. J. Artif. Intell. Tools **23**(01), 1440001 (2014)
40. Cook, D.J., Crandall, A.S., Thomas, B.L., Krishnan, N.C.: CASAS: a smart home in a box. Computer **46**(7), 62–69 (2013)
41. Center for Advanced Studies in Adaptive Systems, "Datasets," WSU CASAS, 2014.
42. Parisa Rashidi: Ambient intelligence datasets. http://www.cise.ufl.edu/~prashidi/Datasets/ambientIntelligence.html (2013). Accessed 18 Sept 2015

Chapter 6
Discussion

Abstract This chapter briefly discusses the anticipated future challenges within the field of monitoring older adults and provides a number of future research directions. Some of the most notable challenges are lack of publically available datasets, poor measurement accuracy of sensors, user-centered design barriers, and user acceptability for monitoring. We try to draw attention to the importance of acquiring objective information of older patients' health conditions by applying appropriate sensor technology for automated monitoring, which we covered in the previous chapters of this book. As possible future research directions, we draw attention to the necessary research in the fields of sensor fusion and machine learning for detecting various health-threatening events and conditions in older population.

Keywords Future challenges • Research directions • User-centered design • Acceptability • Time delays • Sampling limitations • Datasets • Accuracy • Taxonomy

The need for objective measurements of older patients' conditions in the home environment is a critical ingredient of assessment before institutionalization. In the absence of such measurements, the relationship between certain activities or inactivity, for example, cannot be related to the appearance of a specific health-threatening event or condition. To date, there is no routine procedure available to measure activity in a home setting. Attempts to overcome this have predominantly employed archaic methods using observations and surveys, which are susceptible to observation and interpretation bias, as well as cannot be directly applied to those patients who are living alone.

6.1 Future Challenges

6.1.1 Defining Taxonomy

In-home activity monitoring initially requires definitions of activities, level of correspondence between activities, and an established relationship model between the activities. These can be achieved by defining taxonomy of activities systematically.

J. Klonovs et al., *Distributed Computing and Monitoring Technologies for Older Patients*, SpringerBriefs in Computer Science,
DOI 10.1007/978-3-319-27024-1_6

Unfortunately, except the work of [1], which manually defined taxonomy of some daily living activities, no systematic study was accomplished in order to define the taxonomy of daily living activities in a private home.

6.1.2 Lack of Publicly Available Datasets

The availability of public datasets is necessary to compare the methods proposed to solve similar problems. However, a few datasets are available in public to assess the methods proposed in the literature. Moreover, the available datasets have the limitation of the experimental setup and standard quality assurance. It is also observed from our book that most of the previously proposed methods used custom datasets instead of publicly available datasets, and furthermore, many of the authors did not make their dataset publicly available due to privacy policies. Thus, there is a need of regulatory initiatives, which would lessen the hurdles for the researchers' community to access and publish datasets necessary for solving the emerging healthcare problems.

6.1.3 Inefficiency of Health-Threat Detection Technologies

As discussed in our book, a number of health-threat detection methods have been proposed; however the false alarm rates from the methods are still questionable. Moreover, majority of authors used their own custom datasets to generate experimental results for their proposed methods and thus provided less room for comparison between different methods.

6.1.4 Sampling Limitations and Time Delays in Monitoring

Every sensor has temporal sampling limitations, which need to be considered. Every measurement process involves some time delays in data capture, which depend on various factors, such as location of sensors and sensing modality. In general, sensor signals are noisy and thus require digital filtering, which causes certain time delays as well. Furthermore, delays in sensor signals may or may not be constant [2]. If the sampling frequency is too low or irregular, interpolating the measurements reliably over time might not be feasible depending on a given problem. Estimating eventual time delays between irregularly sampled time series is crucial for avoiding possible data processing and interpretation errors. For scenarios, where multiple sensors are used, time synchronization among all sensors is necessary to enable fusion of sensory data, which can be increasingly difficult, because different time delays in data acquisition, transmission, and processing may be present. In addition, the time lag between sampling and obtaining the analysis results may be ranging from a matter of milliseconds to several hours, which can be a significant problem if the situation requires immediate decision concerning patient's health.

Choosing an optimal sampling frequency in order to provide sufficient resolution for detecting a certain health threat is generally not a trivial task. Some sensor types may have an advantage over other sensors in terms of resolution and detection times for certain health threats. It can be discussed at length whether monitoring a certain parameter is necessary for a given problem, while taking into account various trade-offs between sample sizes, measurement costs, detection accuracy, privacy, and comfortability of monitoring. Understanding these trade-offs requires further research. Furthermore, adaptive sampling techniques might be useful for scenarios, where it does not make sense to continuously measure a certain parameter rather than to take a sample once in a while or only when the risk of a health threat is detected by analyzing other parameters. Such approach may potentially improve energy efficiency, when certain sensors can be in sleep mode and are set active only when there is an identified need for using them in time.

Another area of great importance, which we did not have the space to cover, is ICT solutions for the transmission of large data over long distances, which can potentially improve the accessibility of monitoring technologies for those living in rural areas. Network delays in data transmission can have a critical impact on detecting health threats at home. Even for relatively short distances, the network delay problem may present a significant obstacle for monitoring scenarios. One example is the delay in active camera-based systems, which use the pan-tilt-zoom capability of video cameras. Industry standard available cameras exhibit long network delays in executing move instructions. Thus, real-time monitoring and tracking suffer from the camera delays and frequently miss the object of interest during monitoring or tracking. Thus, active research is necessary to address network delay problem as well [3].

6.1.5 Accuracy in Measuring Physiological Parameters

Although a number of innovative methods have been proposed for physiological parameter measurements, for example, automatic heart rate measurement by using facial image or fingertip image from video cameras, the accuracy of such approach is not up to the standard yet, while successful examples were only possible in highly limited lab conditions. Besides, when the facial expression changes or the face moves in the video frames, the accuracy of heart rate estimation decreases significantly. To overcome this problem, the use of quality assessment techniques as an intermediate step between facial detection and relevant feature extraction was recently proposed [4].

6.1.6 User-Centered Design Barriers for Older Adults

Resolving barriers to engagement, participation, and spreading of telemonitoring service programs among older populations is challenging [5]. In [5], authors described the specific issues concerning technological acceptance, human resource development, and collaboration with service systems. They discussed possible strategies and policy implications with regard to human-computer interaction design considerations for telemonitoring of medical and aging conditions of older adults and possible improvements for the access to technology services and additional training for effective use of the technology. However, it can be increasingly challenging to find a balance between user requirements for designing a dedicated technological solution for a specific need of some target patients and for complying such solution with the *Universal Design* principles [6] at the same time. In our view, the concept of *Universal Design* should not be seen as a synonym to *user-centeredness* for designing and applying monitoring technology to older patients; in other words, "one size fits all" cannot be used in this context. It is important to have end-users involved in the process of designing, testing, and evaluating the monitoring technologies [7].

6.1.7 User Acceptability in Monitoring

As stated in [8], accepting monitoring systems in a person's home, especially when it is the home of an older person, is very difficult. This is due to the fact that people do not want to be monitored for privacy concerns, even if this is necessary for assisted living. However, if it is possible to provide high data and privacy protection by other means, then the acceptability can be increased, as discussed in [9]. Therefore, privacy is a crucial consideration for the design and implementation of monitoring technologies.

6.2 Future Research Directions

First, as a prerequisite to further research in this field, a direct involvement of various end-users is needed, including healthy, vulnerable, and acutely ill older adults, as well as their family members and healthcare staff, to ensure the quality and applicability of monitoring technologies in real-life settings. Further research is necessary that can contribute to creation of a systematic guideline for developing benchmarking datasets for the topics covered in Chap. 3. For collecting new datasets, it would be important to use multiple sensor categories for collecting a wide diversity of measurable parameters (see Sect. 4.1.3) and to apply sensor fusion techniques with a purpose of dealing with uncertainties in detecting individual health threats. For example, those datasets should at least contain both physiological parameters and data about environmental conditions of older adults collected at the same time. More effort should be put on creating and applying generative machine learning methods on these datasets, instead of discriminative methods, with the purpose of detecting new health-threatening events and conditions in older population. Furthermore, the research on machine learning techniques should in principle be done in collaboration with the involved healthcare personnel to ensure that the algorithms are properly understood. For this reason, further research on graphical models and incorporating them into end user interfaces is expected to be beneficial. For future studies, it is important to clearly communicate the limitations of the developed systems and constrains of their evaluation results. Last but not least, further research is needed to find the balance between privacy constrains of data collection and what data is a strict requirement for successful monitoring of specific geriatric conditions.

References

1. Pirsiavash, H., Ramanan, D.: Detecting activities of daily living in first-person camera views. In: 2012 IEEE Conference on Computer Vision and Pattern Recognition (CVPR), pp. 2847–2854 (2012)
2. Keenan, D.B., Mastrototaro, J.J., Voskanyan, G., Steil, G.M.: Delays in minimally invasive continuous glucose monitoring devices: a review of current technology. J. Diabetes Sci. Technol. **3**(5), 1207–1214 (2009)
3. Ke, S.R., Thuc, H., Lee, Y.J., Hwang, J.N., Yoo, J.H., Choi, K.H.: A review on video-based human activity recognition. Computers **2**(2), 88–131 (2013)
4. Haque, M.A., Nasrollahi, K., Moeslund, T.B.: Constructing facial expression log from video sequences using face quality assessment. Presented at the International Conference on Computer Vision Theory and Applications, Lisbon, Portugal (2014)
5. Chen, H., Levkoff, S.E.: Delivering telemonitoring care to digitally disadvantaged older adults: human-computer interaction (HCI) design recommendations. In: Zhou, J., Salvendy, G. (eds.) Human aspects of IT for the aged population. Design for everyday life, pp. 50–60. Springer International Publishing, (2015)
6. Cook, A.M., Polgar, J.M.: Assistive Technologies: Principles and Practice. Elsevier Health Sciences (2014)
7. Rodeschini, G.: Gerotechnology: a new kind of care for aging? An analysis of the relationship between older people and technology. Nurs. Health Sci. **13**(4), 521–528 (2011)
8. Rashidi, P., Mihailidis, A.: A survey on ambient-assisted living tools for older adults. IEEE J. Biomed. Health Inform. **17**(3), 579–590 (2013)
9. Cardinaux, F., Bhowmik, D., Abhayaratne, C., Hawley, M.S.: Video based technology for ambient assisted living: a review of the literature. J. Ambient Intell. Smart Environ. **3**(3), 253–269 (2011)

Chapter 7
Conclusion

Abstract This chapter concludes the book by summarizing the current status and visions for research and developments in the cross-disciplinary field of monitoring older populations.

Keywords Data quality • eHealth • IT literacy • Older populations • Benchmarking • Further research • Non-intrusiveness • Machine learning • Smart-homes • Telemonitoring • Ambient intelligence • Ambient-assisted living • Gerotechnology • Aging-in-place technology • Healthcare • Long-term care • Welfare systems

Common data quality standards for patient databases and datasets need to be developed, because currently little is known about how to organize and store data from monitored older patients in an efficient way, which is a prerequisite for learning. Also benchmarking techniques for testing the performance of machine learning techniques on these datasets are currently lacking. As the number of databases and datasets with diverse data about older patients at home is very limited but is on the rise, we are only at the beginning of understanding and analyzing these data. Though, the number of possible applications is high. As long as no single machine learning technique proved to be substantially superior to others for some given task, it would be wise to run multiple algorithms whenever possible for objective comparison of these learning approaches.

The described technological applications are mainly aimed at older adults, and as mentioned earlier, it is of utmost importance to understand the enormous heterogeneity of the older populations. This heterogeneity has the effect that there is no such thing as "one size fits all." Also, *eHealth* technology has to be adaptable to the needs of the individual older adults, i.e., to his or hers cognitive, physical, emotional, and societal skills as well as the environment. The heterogeneity is further enlarged by the differences in IT skills and competencies of older adults both today and in the near future, as some countries already today have a high proportion of IT literate older adults, while other countries have a majority of older adults with low educational attainment and IT-illiteracy. A further constraint is that, while the most remote and rural areas would benefit a lot in using *eHealth*, these areas are usually also those with the most poorly developed IT-infrastructure, a fact that emphasizes the challenges of using *eHealth* in the health monitoring of

J. Klonovs et al., *Distributed Computing and Monitoring Technologies for Older Patients*, SpringerBriefs in Computer Science,
DOI 10.1007/978-3-319-27024-1_7

older adults. Hopefully, innovative solutions for the transmission of large data over long distances will soon come and thereby would add to some of the solutions to challenges of aging societies.

Indeed, the room for innovative solutions in the area of monitoring older adults at home environment is very large, and a lot of improvements of existing solutions can be made. Non-intrusiveness and noninvasiveness of sensor technology will likely be the key factor for successful application. Smaller and cheaper types of sensors, such as piezoresistive and piezoelectric textile sensors, will have the advantage for becoming a part of daily life of older adults, because they have a better potential to be embedded in garments and furniture with prospect of being comfortable and reusable. In terms of advances in software solutions, various machine learning techniques have shown a great potential towards more reliable detection of health-threatening situations and conditions of older adults. There is a large research potential for the interplay of unsupervised and supervised learning, where there is only a small amount of labeled data and a large amount of unlabeled data available, because for many of the patient-at-home scenarios data labeling can be expensive and time consuming. Furthermore, combining the available knowledge from the research results of the various cross-disciplinary fields of smart-homes, telemonitoring, ambient intelligence, ambient-assisted living, gerotechnology, aging-in-place technology, and others, which we have mentioned in this book, can boost the further development of technological monitoring solutions for healthcare, long-term care, and welfare systems to better meet the needs of aging populations.

Printed in the United States
By Bookmasters